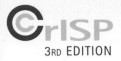

3RD EDITION

# Care of the
# Critically Ill Surgical Patient®

EDITED BY IAN LOFTUS

First published in Great Britain in 1999 by Hodder Arnold
Second edition 2003
This third edition published in 2010 by
Hodder Arnold, an imprint of Hodder Education,
part of Hachette Livre UK, 338 Euston Road, London NW1 3BH

http://www.hodderarnold.com

Whilst the advice and information in this book are believed to
be true and accurate at the date of going to press, neither the
author[s] nor the publisher can accept any legal responsibility or
liability for any errors or omissions that may be made. In particular
(but without limiting the generality of the preceding disclaimer)
every effort has been made to check drug dosages; however it is
still possible that errors have been missed. Furthermore, dosage
schedules are constantly being revised and new side-effects
recognized. For these reasons the reader is strongly urged to
consult the drug companies' printed instructions before administering
any of the drugs recommended in this book.

*British Library Cataloguing in Publication Data*
A catalogue record for this book is available from the British Library

*Library of Congress Cataloging-in-Publication Data*
A catalog record for this book is available from the Library of Congress

ISBN-13    978-0-340-98724-7

2 3 4 5 6 7 8 9 10

Commissioning Editor: Gavin Jamieson
Cover Designer: Chatland Design

Typeset in Rotis Family 10pt by Chatland Design
Printed in Italy

What do you think about this book? Or any other Hodder Arnold title?
Please visit our website: www.hodderarnold.com

# CONTENTS

*Success depends upon attention to detail*

Joseph Lister 1827–1912

## CONTRIBUTORS TO THE 3RD EDITION

**Mr Ian Loftus** BSc MB ChB MD FRCS
*Consultant Vascular Surgeon and Reader
in Vascular Science, St George's Hospital, London
Editor and Critical Care Tutor,
The Royal College of Surgeons of England*

**Mr Iain Anderson** FRCS
*Consultant Surgeon, Hope Hospital, Salford*

**Dr Daniele Bryden** FRCA
*Consultant Anaesthetist, Northern General Hospital*

**Mr Francis Calder** FRCSEd
*Consultant Transplant Surgeon, Guy's Hospital,
London*

**Dr Joseph Cosgrove** FRCA
*Consultant Anaesthetist, Freeman Hospital,
Newcastle*

**Dr Sarah Gillis** FRCA
*Consultant Anaesthetist, Whittington Hospital,
London*

**Dr Jonathan Goodall** FRCA
*Consultant in Intensive Care, Hope Hospital, Salford*

**Mr John Jameson** FRCS
*Consultant General Surgeon,
Leicester General Hospital*

**Mr Brian Johnson** FRCS
*Consultant Vascular Surgeon, Hull Royal Infirmary*

**Mr Keith Jones** FRCS
*Consultant Vascular Surgeon, St George's Hospital,
London*

**Dr Philip Newman** FRCA
*Consultant Anaesthetist, St George's Hospital,
London*

**Mr Declan O'Brian** FRCA
*Consultant Anaesthetist, Cork University Hospital*

**Professor Rob Sayers** FRCS
*Consultant Vascular Surgeon,
Leicester Royal Infirmary*

**Mr Mark Taylor** PhD FRCS
*Consultant General and Hepatobiliary Surgeon,
Mater Informorum Hospital, Belfast*

## CONTRIBUTORS TO THE 2ND EDITION

Mr G L Carlson FRCS
Dr M Hunter FRCAS
Dr B Riley FRCA
Professor B J Rowlands FRCS
Dr G B Smith FRCA
Professor M M Thompson FRCS

## CONTRIBUTORS TO THE 1ST EDITION

Dr T N Appleyard
Professor K CH Fearon
Mr D R Griffin
Professor D J Leaper
Dr G Ramsay
Mr R C G Russell
Professor J M Ryan
Dr A I K Short
Dr S W Turner
Dr R G Wheatley

## ACKNOWLEDGEMENTS

**Mr Adrian Anthony** MB BS FRACS
*Consultant Surgeon,*
*Queen Elizabeth Hospital, Australia*

**Mr Adam Brownsell**
*Publisher,*
*The Royal College of Surgeons of England*

**Miss Emma Church**
*Development and QA Coordinator,*
*The Royal College of Surgeons of England*

# FOREWORD TO 1st EDITION

On Saturday 15 April 1989, at a football match in the English city of Sheffield, an incident occurred in a tightly packed crowd which resulted in 96 mainly young people being crushed to death with many others seriously injured. The name of the football ground, Hillsborough, has become embedded in the English language as being synonymous with a major civilian disaster associated with needless loss of life. It would be difficult to see how anything positive could emerge from such a tragedy but there is a precedent, admittedly on a much smaller scale.

In 1976, in rural Nebraska, USA, a plane being piloted by an orthopaedic surgeon crashed. One of the six occupants was killed instantly and four were critically injured. The primary care received by the injured was judged by the doctors at the admitting hospital, and the orthopaedic surgeon himself, to be less than ideal. As a result the local surgeons decided that they should take some action to establish innovative training courses to help those unused to managing the seriously injured to deal with such cases. Thus arose the now well-recognised and respected Advanced Trauma Life Support (ATLS®) courses which use simulation and scene setting to mimic major injury and to improve the quality and realism or training.

In 1988 ATLS® was introduced into the United Kingdom by The Royal College of Surgeons of England and became instantly popular with all those tasked with the management of the seriously injured, and there is no doubt that ATLS® techniques were used at Hillsborough and may well have prevented an even higher death rate. Although difficult to prove scientifically, there is virtually universal agreement that ATLS® courses have improved care and contributed to the lowering of the death rate after road traffic accidents which has become such a marked feature of United Kingdom accident statistics of recent years. ATLS® however, deals only with the early stage of injury and there is undoubtedly a need for improvement in the management of that critical period following injury, during critical surgical illness, or after major surgery where patients may be in intensive therapy or high dependency units.

The educational techniques used in ATLS® are equally applicable in critical care training. Iain Anderson and his colleagues, with the help of the Education Department at The Royal College of Surgeons of England and the support of the Hillsborough Charity, have produced a course similar in concept to ATLS® and using its techniques, dealing with the management of the critically ill surgical patient. This book is produced in a format that will enable the text to be used either independently or alongside the course. This innovative approach has the potential for improving the care of critically ill patients in the same manner and to the same degree as that achieved by ATLS®.

The book deals concisely and clearly with the whole range of issues associated with the critically ill, including the management of the psychological problems which were such an issue after Hillsborough. The surgical trainees who undergo this course and read this textbook will have restored to them the confidence once felt by all surgical trainees in the management of the critically ill. This confidence was based on the famous textbook by the American surgeon Francis Moore, *The Metabolic Care of the Surgical Patient*, a book that is widely accepted as being the foundation stone of modern intensive care.

I hope those so tragically bereaved at Hillsborough will regard this book and its accompanying course as a living addition to the more permanent memorial in Liverpool to those who died.

**Sir Miles Irving**
DSc (Hons) MD ChM FRCS FACS (Hon) FMedSci

*Emeritus Professor of Surgery,*
*University of Manchester*

*Chairman of Newcastle upon Tyne Hospitals*
*NHS Trust*

# PREFACE

Surgical training has undergone major changes over the last decade. While hours of duty for doctors in training have been reduced by legislation designed to improve patient care, so clinical exposure has been reduced and traditional surgical teams fragmented. One could argue that modern day surgical trainees are under more pressure than ever before, despite the reduction in working hours. Trainees often feel disengaged from their trainers, and their patients, due to shift working patterns that are disruptive to traditional training methods. Moreover, because of a lack of clinical exposure, they often feel unprepared to deal with emergencies and the care of the critically ill patient.

The Care of the Critically Ill Surgical Patient (CCrISP) course remains a valuable adjunct to traditional ward training and continues to provide young surgeons with the structure and confidence they require to safely and effectively care for their patients on the ward and in theatre. This third edition of the course, originally launched by Iain Anderson and colleagues in 1996, remains true to the original aims to take responsibility for critically ill surgical patients, to 'predict and prevent' problems that patients might encounter while in hospital, to function well within the surgical team and communicate effectively with colleagues from other disciplines.

The CCrISP course was originally established by a multidisciplinary team of surgeons and anaesthetists with a grant from the Hillsborough football stadium disaster. Many of the original group continue to instruct on the CCrISP course and some have been involved in this latest iteration of the material and manual. The majority of surgical trainees in the UK take the course, available in over 60 centres, and it is compulsory in Australasia. More recently, the START (Systematic Training in Acute Illness Recognition and Treatment) Surgery course has adopted the CCrISP principles successfully for the training of foundation year doctors. A CCrISP Instructor course also runs at The Royal College of Surgeons of England to prepare senior surgeons, who have all taken the CCrISP course during their training, for providing the course nationwide. This continuum of surgical critical care training has been supported generously for many years by Jane and Leon Grant, to whom this third edition is dedicated.

The new edition of the course continues to reinforce the clinical application of the theory base provided in this manual. The manual has been updated significantly, with some chapters removed entirely, replaced with new chapters felt to be more relevant to current surgical trainees. The principles remain the same – to encourage the development of practical skills, improved patient management and the development of interpersonal skills required to work effectively and confidently within a surgical team. The need to master these skills early in training has never been more pressing, given the changes to working patterns and demands on time.

The CCrISP algorithm for simultaneous assessment and resuscitation has become the benchmark for the management of surgical patients and is used by even the most senior, experienced surgeons on a daily basis.

As with previous editions, this review is based on the opinions of a multidisciplinary steering group that has worked tirelessly to ensure that it represents the needs of current surgical trainees. I hope that you will find it instructive and beneficial to the care you provide to your patients.

Ian Loftus

*A stitch in time saves nine*

Traditional

# CCrISP COURSE OBJECTIVES

- Develop the theoretical basis and practical skills necessary to manage the critically ill surgical patient

- Be able to assess critically ill patients accurately and appreciate the value of a system of assessment for the critically ill

- Understand the subtlety and variety of presentation of critical illness and the methods available for improving detection

- Understand the importance of a plan of action in order to achieve clinical progress, accurate diagnosis and early definitive treatment. Be able to formulate a plan of action and involve appropriate assistance in a timely manner

- Appreciate that complications tend to occur in a cascade and realise that prevention of complications is fundamental to successful outcome

- Be aware of the support facilities available and interact with nursing staff, other surgeons and intensivists/anaesthetists, being aware, in particular, of the surgeon's role in the delivery of multidisciplinary care to the critically ill

- Understand the requirements of the patient and his or her relatives during critical illness and be able to inform and support both appropriately.

# ABBREVIATIONS

| | | | | |
|---|---|---|---|---|
| ABG | arterial blood gas | | DPL | diagnostic peritoneal lavage |
| ACE | angiotensin-converting enzyme | | DVT | deep vein thrombosis |
| ACS | acute compartment syndrome | | | |
| ADH | antidiuretic hormone | | ECF | extracellular fluid |
| A&E | accident and emergency | | ECG | electrocardiogram |
| AF | atrial fibrillation | | ECLS | extracorporeal life support |
| AKIN | acute kidney injury network | | EEG | electroencephalogram |
| AP | anteroposterior | | EIA | epidural infusion analgesia |
| ARDS | acute respiratory distress syndrome | | ENT | ear, nose and throat |
| ASB | assisted spontaneous breathing | | ERCP | endoscopic retrograde |
| ATLS® | Advanced Trauma Life Support® | | | cholangiopancreatography |
| AV | atrioventricular | | | |
| | | | FAST | focused abdominal sonography |
| BAL | bronchial alveolar lavage | | | in trauma |
| BBB | bundle branch block | | FBC | full blood count |
| BCAA | branched-chain amino acid | | $FEV_1$ | forced expiratory volume in 1 s |
| BE | base excess | | FRC | functional residual capacity |
| BLS | basic life support | | FTc | corrected flow time |
| BMI | body mass index | | | |
| BSA | body surface area | | GABA | gamma-aminobutyric acid |
| | | | GCS | Glasgow coma scale |
| CCF | congestive cardiac failure | | GI | gastrointestinal |
| CCrISP | Care of the Critically Ill Surgical Patient | | | |
| CI | cardiac index | | HDU | high dependency unit |
| CNS | central nervous system | | HIV | human immunodeficiency virus |
| COAD | chronic obstructive airways disease | | 5-HT | 5-hydroxytrptamine (serotonin) |
| COX-2 | cyclo-oxygenase 2 | | | |
| CPAP | continuous positive airway pressure | | IAP | intra-abdominal pressure |
| CPP | cerebral perfusion pressure | | ICU | intensive care unit |
| CPR | cardiopulmonary resuscitation | | ICP | intracranial pressure |
| CRF | chronic renal failure | | IgE | immunoglobulin E |
| CSM | carotid sinus massage | | IHD | ischaemic heart disease |
| CT | computed tomography | | IVNAA | in vivo neuron activation analysis |
| CTZ | chemoreceptor trigger zone | | IVU | intravenous urogram |
| CVP | central venous pressure | | | |
| CVS | cardiovascular system | | JVP | jugular venous pressure |
| CXR | chest X-ray | | | |

| | | | | |
|---|---|---|---|---|
| LAP | left atrial pressure | | RRT | renal replacement therapy |
| LFT | liver function test | | | |
| LVEDP | left ventricular end diastolic pressure | | SIMV | synchronised intermittent mandatory ventilation |
| LVEDV | left ventricular end diastolic volume | | SIRS | systemic inflammatory response syndrome |
| LVF | left ventricular failure | | SVC | superior vena cava |
| MAP | mean arterial pressure | | SVR | systemic vascular resistance |
| MEWS | modified early warning score | | SVT | supraventricular tachycardia |
| MI | myocardial infarction | | | |
| MOF | multiple organ failure | | TNF | tumour necrosis factor |
| MRI | magnetic resonance imaging | | TOD | trans-oesophageal Doppler |
| MRSA | methicillin-resistant *Staphyloccus aureus* | | | |
| | | | VF | ventriculation fibrillation |
| NCA | nurse-controlled analgesia | | VT | ventricular tachycardia |
| NICE | National Institute for Health and Clinical Excellence | | | |
| NIV | non-invasive ventilation | | WPW | Wolff Parkinson White syndrome |
| NSAID | non-steroidal anti-inflammatory drug | | | |

LAP    left atrial pressure
LFT    liver function test
LVEDP  left ventricular end diastolic pressure
LVEDV  left ventricular end diastolic volume
LVF    left ventricular failure

MAP    mean arterial pressure
MEWS   modified early warning score
MI     myocardial infarction
MOF    multiple organ failure
MRI    magnetic resonance imaging
MRSA   methicillin-resistant *Staphyloccus aureus*

NCA    nurse-controlled analgesia
NICE   National Institute for
       Health and Clinical Excellence
NIV    non-invasive ventilation
NSAID  non-steroidal anti-inflammatory drug

OSA    obstructive sleep apnoea

PA     postero-anterior
PAOP   pulmonary artery occlusion pressure
PAP    pulmonary artery pressure
PCA    patient-controlled analgesia
PCIRV  pressure-controlled inverse
       ratio ventilation
PCV    pressure-controlled ventilation
PCWP   pulmonary capillary wedge pressure
PE     pulmonary embolism
PEEP   positive end expiratory pressure
PEM    protein-energy malnutrition
PiCCO  pulse contour cardiac output with
       dicator dilution
PSV    pressure-support ventilation
PTC    percutaneous trans-hepatic cholangiography
PTSD   post-traumatic stress disorder

RRT    renal replacement therapy

SIMV   synchronised intermittent
       mandatory ventilation
SIRS   systemic inflammatory response
       syndrome
SVC    superior vena cava
SVR    systemic vascular resistance
SVT    supraventricular tachycardia

TNF    tumour necrosis factor
TOD    trans-oesophageal Doppler

VF     ventriculation fibrillation
VT     ventricular tachycardia

WPW    Wolff Parkinson White syndrome

# NORMAL LABORATORY VALUES

| Measurement | Normal range |
| --- | --- |
| Sodium | 135–145 mmol/l |
| Potassium | 3.5–5.0 mmol/l |
| Urea | 3.1–7.9 mmol/l |
| Creatinine | 75–155 µmol/l |
| Total protein | 58–78 g/l |
| Albumin | 34–50 g/l |
| Calcium | 2.12–2.60 mmol/l |
| Phosphate ($PO_4^{3-}$) | 0.80–1.44 mmol/l |
| Bilirubin | 0–19 µmol/l |
| Alkaline phosphatase | 35–120 units/l |
| ALT | 0–45 units/l |
| Creatine kinase | Male: 38–174 units/L | Female: 96–140 units/L |
| Haemoglobin | 13.0–18.0 g/l |
| Platelets | 150–450 x $10^9$/l |
| White cell count | 4.0–11.0 x $10^9$/l |
| Prothrombin time | 11.0–13.0 s |
| APTT | 24–39 s |
| Fibrinogen | 1.5–4.0 g/l |
| pH | 7.35–7.45 |
| $PaCO_2$ | 4.5–5.5 kPa (34–42 mmHg) |
| $PaO_2$ | 11.0–14.0 kPa (83–105 mmHg) |
| $HCO_3^-$ | 24–28 mmol/l |
| Base excess | -2 to +2 mmol/l |
| Lactate | 0.4–1.7 mmol/l |

# 1

# Introduction

Looking after critically ill surgical patients successfully is a major and, at times, stressful part of the surgeon's life. Surgical practice is dynamic and as changes to hospital practice occur, they may help or hinder other aspects of the delivery of care. Some of the current factors are shown in Table 1.1.

## TABLE 1.1

### RISK AND STRESS FACTORS IN SURGICAL CRITICAL CARE

- Ageing population
- Concomitant disease processes
- Complexity of surgery
- Higher standards of monitoring
- Greater number of postoperative interventions and therapies
- Expectations by patients, relatives and staff
- Shortage of permanent and experienced nurses
- Shortened duty hours for junior surgeons and different on-call arrangements

Many surgical patients are old, sick, have undergone major surgery or have had emergency admission. With modern duty arrangements, you will often be responsible for this type of patient from other surgical teams and you may well be on duty with junior and senior staff with whom you only work occasionally. Consequently, the duty surgeon will be faced frequently with critically ill surgical patients with whom they are not familiar. The establishment of high dependency units (HDUs) has been an undoubted advance but not all unwell patients can be cared for there and, in any event, patient care in HDU often remains the

responsibility of the surgical team. Furthermore, to the unfamiliar, the HDU can be a daunting place. The CCrISP programme provides practical training to support the junior doctor who is faced with managing unwell surgical patients today. In particular, it provides a simple, safe and accepted approach with which you can begin to assess and manage every patient you encounter, no matter how complex.

The capacity of surgical patients to withstand surgery and any complications depends on their age, underlying disease process and any co-existing illnesses. Once surgical patients develop multiple organ failure (and hence require intensive care unit [ICU] support), overall mortality can be around 50%. It is clear, therefore, that detecting and treating problems before this stage is reached is much the preferable course of action. Unfortunately, critical surgical illness can often be detected easily only once a relatively advanced stage has been reached. The challenge for all surgeons who deal with patients who may become critically ill is to develop a system of practice which will allow the identification and correction of complications at the earliest stage. Improvements can be achieved through three mechanisms as summarised in Table 1.2.

## TABLE 1.2

### COMPLEMENTARY APPROACHES TO CRITICAL CARE

- Prediction: identifying an at-risk population
- Prevention
- Prompt identification and early adequate treatment

These are complementary and will apply in differing proportions to different patient groups. These strategies are at least as important components of surgical critical care as the heroic, but often unsuccessful, rescue of the patient who has reached a state of extremis.

## AIM OF TRAINING IN SURGICAL CRITICAL CARE

Critical illness begins, is detectable and treatable long before a patient arrives in an ICU with multiple organ failure, and the aim of this manual and its related course, the CCrISP course of The Royal College of Surgeons of England, is to equip you to predict, prevent and treat these patients accordingly. Likewise, it will be difficult to offer best care to emergency cases or to unfit patients upon whom you conduct major surgery without the necessary management skills for ward and HDU practice. Surgical training has traditionally focused on pathology and operative surgical treatment; however, with the advances in critical care techniques and changes in patient demographics, more structured teaching in non-operative management of critically ill patients is essential.

### AIMS OF THE CCrISP COURSE

Improve practical management of critically ill surgical patients
- clinical method
- practical skills
- communication and organisational skills
- focused knowledge.

Too many deaths or unplanned admissions to ICU occur because appropriate, thoughtful and early action was not taken. Studies show that 30–40% of patients admitted to ICU received sub-optimal care on the ward at some stage. Together with the CCrISP course, this book aims to make you think about the ill or potentially ill patient. It will help you identify the patient who may become ill and take the necessary steps to prevent that patient developing complications; to deal with any emergency arising on the ward; to assess and respond to the immediate problem; and to initiate treatment while awaiting specialist help. Following immediate management, you will learn the importance of identifying and correcting the underlying cause. Many adverse episodes can be terminated by the immediate provision of simple support (*e.g.* oxygen, fluids) and by the early attainment of a diagnosis so early definitive treatment can be instituted (*e.g.* antibiotics, provision of usual cardiac medications, drainage of an abscess).

### PRACTICE POINT

*Prompt, simple actions save lives and prevent complications.*

Avoidable problems occur because these simple manoeuvres are not taken or, more commonly, their effectiveness and adequacy is not checked and further effective steps not taken. For example, failure to institute and ensure effective support for an elderly patient with retained pulmonary secretions on a Saturday may result in established pneumonia by Monday morning. Survival may be threatened and length of stay will certainly be prolonged (Case Scenario 1.1).

## CASE SCENARIO 1.1

A 68-year-old man, a smoker with mild chronic airways disease, underwent a laparotomy for a perforated duodenal ulcer on Monday night. An epidural was placed but was removed on day 4 (Friday). He received chest physiotherapy during the week but no specific request was made for weekend treatment. His team was not on call and, as he seemed to be progressing, no formal handover was made. On Saturday afternoon, he was noted to be in pain and to have a tachypnoea. The foundation year doctor was called but was busy and did not see him until 9 a.m. by which time he was pyrexial. A course of ciprofloxacin was prescribed (although none would be available from the pharmacy until 9 a.m.). He was reviewed at the end of the on-call ward round, late Sunday morning, and found to have deteriorated considerably, with pyrexia, dyspnoea and bronchial breathing. He was started on monitored oxygen, nebulisers and urgent chest physiotherapy was arranged, following review of his requirements for analgesia. He took 10 days to get over the pneumonia and his hospital stay was prolonged by about 2 weeks.

### LEARNING POINTS

- the best critical care is simple and preventive – late, heroic interventions are less successful
- prompt, simple actions save lives and prevent complications
- make, use and update action plans
- success depends on attention to detail.

Achieving simple interventions, such as the oxygen, nebulisers and physiotherapy in the case above, requires the same combination of skills as more complex or dramatic episodes in surgical critical care. These include clinical examination, judicious investigation, formulation of a plan of action, institution thereof (including the necessary communication with colleagues and practical techniques), and re-evaluation of the patient with, if necessary, the ability to invoke greater degrees of support at the right time.

These skills, together with relevant practical procedures and the related base knowledge, will be taught and assessed in simulated clinical situations during the CCrISP course, the emphasis throughout being on practical management of common problems. However, there is no reason why you cannot adopt a systematic approach to your own practice directly.

### PRACTICE POINT

*Re-assess!*

*Has your intervention been effective?*

*Further prompt and simple actions may be necessary.*

## WHAT THIS MANUAL IS NOT

Neither this manual nor the CCrISP course will teach you to become a specialist in intensive care! Instead, the main thrust is about prevention of further deterioration through accurate and prompt ASSESSMENT and TREATMENT to avoid complications on the ward and in HDU. However, there does exist a considerable overlap between the practical skills and approaches to care seen on ICU and in the surgical HDU and junior surgeons benefit greatly from a period spent working on ICU. Surgeons must be aware of the nature and principles of intensive care, the support available there and the time when such support should be sought. They must also be aware of the limitations of ICU and the nature of support which the surgical team must provide to the ICU team when their patients are being treated on ICU. During your training, you will need to develop an appreciation of the surgical needs of patients in ICU, the difficulties of assessment there and the impact of ICU care on your patients and their disease processes. Following discharge from ICU, a further range of skills is necessary to ensure that the patient does not fall into the trap of early deterioration and re-admission to ICU. These topics will be dealt with and will contribute towards making you a better practitioner of surgical critical care.

This manual takes a practical, management-orientated approach to critical care. It is not designed to be a comprehensive text of surgical critical care and you may wish to supplement your reading from such a text, particularly for membership examinations.

## CONTINUUM OF CARE

In fact, there is a continuum of care from the ICU through HDU and ward to the community and each provides different attributes of importance to successful surgical care. Compared with surgical wards, the HDU is an area of enhanced nurse to patient ratio (1:2), with appropriate monitoring (arterial, CVP, pulse oximetry, heart rate) equipment and accumulated nursing expertise in both critical illness and specialist surgical care. Patients are usually within 24–72 hours of operation and either at high risk of complications or have developed a complication or impairment of vital organ function on account of their illness, surgery or co-existing medical disease. Some HDUs will manage patients with single organ failure but the main aim is to detect and prevent further deterioration.

By way of contrast, ICU offers more intensive nursing ratios, monitoring and support, and care is usually directed by intensive care medical staff in collaboration with the patient's surgical team. Here, failed organ systems can be supported by complex interventions (*e.g.* ventilation, high dose or multiple inotrope therapy, haemofiltration or dialysis). ICU staff may be less experienced than their HDU counterparts in the surgical aspects of management of patients following complex procedures.

Although the precise profile of patients in different critical care units will vary between hospitals, you should note that many patients will require surgical and intensive care type input whichever type of bed they are in – surgeons have a role to play in the care of patients on ICU and ICU staff often help manage patients on the ward. The proportion of care needed from each team will vary with time and with the patients' immediate needs (Fig. 1.1). HDU occupies a middle ground in terms of the balance between management of surgical problems and the management of systemic or multi-organ problems.

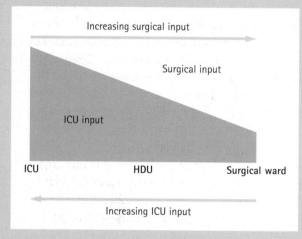

Figure 1.1 **Changing requirements for critical support in surgical patients.**

Special surgical units (*e.g.* transplant units) offer varying combinations of facilities. Assessing and managing patients there will require specialist knowledge and techniques but most of the immediate management relies on the same basic principles. Indeed, many complex problems in critical care can be broken down, assessed and treated in a similar manner.

## THE PATIENTS TO BE CONSIDERED

Situations in which patients are considered at risk or that may increase risk are summarised in Table 1.3. In caring for critically ill surgical patients, three categories of patients can be discerned:
- the routine pre-operative patient
- the emergency admission
- the ward patient.

### TABLE 1.3

**Patients at risk**
- Emergencies
- Elderly
- Co-existing disease processes
- Non-progressing patient
- Severity of acute illness or magnitude of operation
- Massive transfusion
- Re-bleeding
- Failure/delay to diagnose and treat underlying problem
- Already developed another complication
- Established shock state

**Practices that increase risk**
- Incomplete or infrequent assessment
- Failure to act on abnormal findings
- Failure to ensure that interventions have been successful
- Failure of continuity of care (poor communication)
- Failure of nursing support (insufficient numbers or expertise) – wrong ward

*Pre-operative patient*
Patients on steroids for severe chronic airways disease, for example, present obvious risks. Here, a balance must be struck between necessity of operation and the individual risks. Careful specialist and anaesthetic assessment will be needed, if not already obtained, and plans will need to be made for postoperative care. Less obvious problems may act synergistically but a similar approach can minimise their effect (see Case Scenario 1.2).

*The emergency admission*
Emergency admissions present with a wide variety of underlying diseases and an equal spectrum of co-morbid conditions ranging from the unrecognised (*e.g.* occult ischaemic heart disease) to the obvious (*e.g.* anticoagulation), which complicates matters. Many patients undergoing emergency major surgery are inherently unstable and easy prey to further complications. Preventing these begins by achieving prompt and effective resuscitation and surgery – no easy matter in an elderly group presenting out of normal working hours. Anaesthesia removes vascular tone and can cause catastrophic hypotension in the hypovolaemic patient. It is obvious that you cannot do the laparotomy on the patient with peritonitis until he or she is resuscitated but a patient with a fractured neck of femur also requires careful resuscitation. On the other hand, you must identify the bleeding patients who need simultaneous surgery and resuscitation. Co-ordinating appropriate care following surgery, especially out of routine hours, can tax your organisational and communication skills. Clear guidelines must be given to nursing staff and regular medical review undertaken.

## CASE SCENARIO 1.2

Take, for example, the patient for inguinal hernia repair who appears fit but who has left BBBV, a smoker's cough, mild alcoholic liver disease and prostatism. After operation, a predictable chain of minor events may ultimately prove fatal: simple hernia repair leads to urinary retention; subsequent urine infection contributes to a confusional state; failure of expectoration causes atelectasis, then a chest infection; underlying ischaemic heart disease cannot cope with hypoxia. The patient 'suddenly' arrests on day 3 on the short stay ward.

Much of this could have been and should have been predicted. A downward spiral starts with the requirement for a urinary catheter. The significant premorbid conditions contribute to the rapid and relentless deterioration which ultimately leads to the patient's demise.

### LEARNING POINT
- It is crucial to predict and prevent problems, consider the pros and cons of surgery in each individual case, and optimise patients appropriately if surgery is essential.

## The Ward Patient

### The routine ward round

On business ward rounds, you will review all your patients; in fact, this is probably the most important way in which you practise good critical care. By conducting a logical and thorough round, you can prevent or identify many problems and get them corrected before they cause significant upset. The system of assessment and formulation of management plans described in the next chapter applies to these patients every bit as much as to those who are obviously unwell.

### The ward patient with complications

Patients who develop obvious complications present similar challenges to the emergency admissions – the major pitfall being a failure to take further prompt action when initial interventions are not sufficiently successful.

More difficult are patients who 'fail to progress'. Here, there is usually an underlying problem eluding detection. These patients are often elderly; the recognition of subtle signs can lead to appropriate action preventing major problems arising as indicated in Case Scenario 1.2 above.

## METHOD OF APPROACH

Basic surgical trainees are essentially data gatherers – they pass information to seniors. As you progress in seniority, your role changes. You will shortly become a senior trainee, where you will be much more of a decision maker. You will make critical decisions constantly – on ward rounds or about emergencies – which will have a direct bearing on patient outcome. Of course, you will have senior colleagues with whom to discuss things; nevertheless, there is a marked change in role and responsibility at this stage. Using the skills and approaches described in this manual and on the CCrISP course will help you appreciate some of the changes you need to develop. These will aid the change, when it comes, to be less stressful and more successful for all.

All clinicians find the management of emergencies stressful at times and this is usually made worse by a lack of information (about the patient, their diseases or recent events), disorganisation and initial lack of appreciation of the severity of the situation. You will, by now, have experienced episodes in your own practice of critical illness that were not managed as well as they might have been – it is useful at this stage to reflect on the reasons why those sub-optimal events occurred.

The aim now is to build on your present knowledge and experience – to train you to think, to be in command of any situation by rapidly assessing the situation and the patient, responding to the immediate problem and initiating treatment. Certain simple immediate thoughts can help set your assessment off on the right foot (Table 1.4).

## TABLE 1.4

### THINKING ON THE RUN

**Think early** – when the phone call comes
- instructions to caller
- what do I know about ...?
- what will I do when I arrive?

**Think basics** – when I arrive
- check and secure the ABCs
- what system fails?
- what observations are available?
- what observations can I make quickly?

**Think simply**
- how quickly must I act?
- do I have a diagnosis?
- how will I get that diagnosis safely?
- what help do I need?

### THINK THEN ACT

## SUMMARY

- Preventing deterioration is more effective than attempting salvage at a later stage
- Surgical critical care includes prediction and prevention of problems as well as investigation and intervention in the acutely unwell
- There is a continuum in surgical critical care extending from the ward level (prediction, prevention) to HDU and upwards to integrate with intensive care
- Simple logical thought and actions will often be effective.

The CCrISP programme will emphasise certain quite basic clinical and scientific concepts: those that clinicians experienced in this field employ in front-line practice. Above all, it will help you think straight when you are under pressure in the clinical arena. It will provide you with mechanisms that will facilitate successful care, the most important of which is a systematic means to assess a critically ill surgical patient. Until now, you will have approached problems by taking a detailed history and then examining the patient. However, critically ill patients require a system that lets you identify and treat problems rapidly, according to priority and as you further assess the patient. This approach is detailed in the next chapter.

# 2

Assessment of
the critically ill
surgical patient

**OBJECTIVES**

This chapter will help you to:

- assess and manage critically ill patients systematically
- recognise the critically ill patient who must undergo simultaneous examination and resuscitation when first seen
- recognise that examination and resuscitation must be performed in a systematic manner treating life-threatening problems in the order of their threat to life
- be aware of the importance of identifying and correcting the underlying abnormality
- formulate daily management plans for patients on critical care units.

## INTRODUCTION

Surgical patients requiring critical care fall into two broad groups.

First, there are those who are acutely unwell, having been newly admitted or having suffered an acute deterioration on the ward. These patients require simultaneous resuscitation, diagnosis and then definitive treatment.

Second, there are those already on the ward or within HDU who require re-evaluation and formulation of a management plan on at least a twice-daily basis. Here, the aim is to ensure that the patient is progressing, *i.e.* getting better. It is better to prevent morbidity by detecting problems as early as possible; failure to progress is an important sign that an incipient problem

is present. If you fail to diagnose and treat that problem until it has produced a major deterioration in the patient's condition, then the patient's likelihood of survival is dramatically reduced.

The approach to the assessment of the sick surgical patient should be systematic to ensure that life-threatening or potentially life-threatening conditions and important aspects of care are not overlooked. Employing a system regularly ensures that you will use it when you are under pressure. The CCrISP system of assessment is shown in Fig. 2.1. It is the system that many experienced doctors use. The same system is used for all patients, whether stable or unstable.

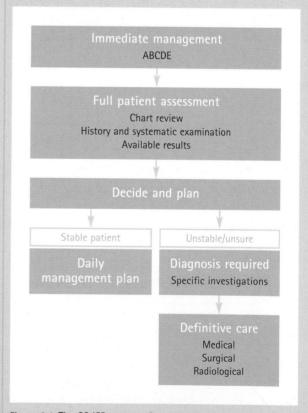

Figure 2.1 The CCrISP system of assessment.

## IMMEDIATE ASSESSMENT AND TREATMENT OF THE ACUTELY ILL PATIENT

When assessing the acutely ill patient, your goal is to determine what is making the patient ill and, having identified any life-threatening problem, to treat it immediately. Life-threatening illnesses kill in a predictable and reproducible pattern. When viewed in isolation, a disease process that produces an obstructed airway will kill more quickly than one which only produces direct lung dysfunction, that, in turn, kills more quickly than isolated haemorrhage or cardiac dysfunction. Many critically ill surgical patients have linked abnormalities of more than one vital system. Hence, it is important not to be distracted by obvious, but minor, factors and to assess and treat problems systematically.

## IMMEDIATE MANAGEMENT

A – Airway assessment and treatment
B – Breathing assessment and treatment
C – Circulation assessment and treatment
D – Dysfunction of the CNS
E – Exposure of the patient sufficient for full assessment and treatment

This process prioritises the order in which assessment and treatment is carried out; although represented as a sequence, such information can often be obtained virtually simultaneously. For example, the patient's response to the question 'How are you?' can be very revealing! If the patient is able to reply in a coherent manner, this suggests that, at least for the moment, he or she is in control of their airway sufficiently to allow an adequate intake of breath, adequate respiratory function to produce oxygen transfer, adequate circulatory function to perfuse the brain and adequate CNS function to formulate a reply. While this is encouraging, it does not release you from the need to perform a detailed assessment of each of the ABCDE components of the immediate assessment.

### PRACTICE POINT

*Be alert to the risks of hepatitis and HIV.*

Always be alert to the risks of blood-borne diseases – in almost all emergencies there is time and facility to adopt safety measures.

### A – AIRWAY

Recognition that airway obstruction is present is based on a simple 'Look, Listen and Feel' clinical assessment, with immediate treatment if there is airway compromise.

- LOOK for the presence of central cyanosis, obstructed 'see-saw' pattern of respiration or abdominal breathing, use of accessory muscles of respiration, tracheal tug, alteration of level of consciousness and any obvious obstruction by foreign body or vomitus
- LISTEN for abnormal sounds such as grunting, snoring, gurgling, hoarseness or stridor
- FEEL for air flow on inspiration and expiration
- TREAT – If objective signs of airway obstruction are present, the immediate goals are to obtain and secure the airway to provide for adequate oxygenation and prevent hypoxic brain damage. Administer high flow oxygen (12–15 l/min, preferably humidified, via a reservoir bag).

Often, only simple methods are required to obtain an airway such as chin lift or jaw thrust to open the airway, suction to remove secretions and either the insertion of an oral Guedel airway (if tolerated) or a soft nasopharyngeal airway (if the gag reflex is present).

If such methods are unsuccessful, a definitive airway (an endotracheal or cuffed tube secured in the trachea) is required. Endotracheal tubes may be passed orally or nasally but the oral route with the larynx visualised by direct laryngoscopy is the most usual choice. This should not be attempted by the untrained; in almost all circumstances, the help of an anaesthetist should be obtained without delay if a secured tube is required. If the patient is in extremis, this may be accomplished without the use of drugs. If the patient is responsive and endotracheal intubation is indicated, you must seek help from an anaesthetist. Always maintain oxygenation throughout airway manoeuvres. Attempts at intubation without first pre-oxygenating the patient are futile and dangerous. If endotracheal intubation is unsuccessful, a surgical airway should be performed: cricothyroidotomy is the technique of choice but, again, this should not be attempted by the untrained.

Remember that patients can be maintained with an airway, plus bag and mask ventilation as required, while waiting for the anaesthetist – this is often a better option for the non-expert, particularly within hospital where skilled help is usually rapidly available.

*Protect the airway*
Patients who are not fully conscious may have an airway that they cannot protect and is only patent intermittently. These patients may tolerate and benefit from airway manoeuvres while the cause of their reduced conscious level is addressed.

Although unusual in the non-trauma situation, if there is a risk of co-existing pathology of the cervical spine, all airway manoeuvres should be performed while maintaining manual in-line immobilisation of the cervical spine.

> **PRACTICE POINT**
> *Get help from an anaesthetist early to secure a compromised airway.*

**B – BREATHING**
Objective evidence of respiratory distress or inadequate ventilation can also be determined using the clinical 'Look, Listen and Feel' technique, followed by immediate treatment of life-threatening conditions:

- LOOK for central cyanosis, use of accessory muscles of respiration, respiratory rate, equality and depth of respiration, sweating, raised JVP, patency of any chest drains and the presence of any paradoxical abdominal movement. Note the inspired oxygen concentration ($FiO_2$) and saturation if pulse oximetry is in use but remember that pulse oximetry does not detect hypercarbia
- LISTEN for noisy breathing, clearance of secretions by coughing, ability of patient to talk in complete sentences (evidence of confusion or decreased level of consciousness may indicate hypoxia or hypercarbia, respectively), change in percussion note and auscultate for abnormal breath sounds, heart sounds and rhythm

- FEEL for equality of chest movement, position of trachea, the presence of surgical emphysema or crepitus, paradoxical respiration and tactile vocal fremitus if indicated. Percuss the chest superiorly and laterally. Abdominal distension may limit diaphragmatic movement and should be looked for as part of respiratory assessment
- TREAT – The precise resuscitative treatment will be determined by the cause of the respiratory embarrassment and will be discussed later in the chapter on respiratory failure (Chapter 4). During the immediate assessment, you should specifically look for signs of the immediately life-threatening conditions: tension pneumothorax, massive haemothorax, open pneumothorax, flail chest and cardiac tamponade should be identified and treated accordingly without delay. Consider also the diagnoses of bronchial obstruction, bronchoconstriction, pulmonary embolism, cardiac failure (see C – Circulation) and unconsciousness (see D – Dysfunction of the nervous system). Simple manoeuvres such as sitting the patient up can help. However, if the patient is tiring to the point of incipient respiratory arrest, assisting ventilation by bag/mask is obligatory, in conjunction with whatever airway manoeuvres have been necessary, until help arrives.

## C – CIRCULATION

Hypovolaemia should always be considered to be the primary cause of circulatory dysfunction in the surgical patient until proven otherwise. Haemorrhage (overt or covert) must be rapidly excluded. Furthermore, unless there are obvious signs of cardiogenic shock (raised JVP particularly), you should regard any patient who is cool and tachycardic to have hypovolaemic shock, so

establish and secure adequate venous access with at least one large (16G) cannula, send blood off for cross-matching and other routine tests, and initiate appropriate fluid replacement. Start with a rapid fluid challenge of 10 ml/kg of warmed crystalloid in the normotensive patient or 20 ml/kg if the patient is hypotensive. You should be more tentative in patients with known heart failure, starting with an initial bolus of 5 ml/kg, unless you suspect that their current problem is pulmonary oedema. Closer monitoring may be needed in these patients.

Having identified and treated airway and breathing abnormalities that can compromise the circulation, life-threatening circulatory dysfunction is recognised by looking for:

- reduced peripheral perfusion (pallor, coolness, collapsed or underfilled veins – remember blood pressure is often normal in the shocked patient)
- obvious external haemorrhage from either wounds or drains
- evidence of concealed haemorrhage: (i) thoracic or abdominal, even when an empty drain is present; (ii) into the gut or from pelvic or femoral fractures; or (iii) alteration of level of consciousness secondary to cerebral under-perfusion.

Initially, you should assess perfusion rather than blood pressure and institute management based on your findings as a priority. Check the blood pressure at an early point; it can often be preserved in a patient with significant circulatory problems. Marked hypotension is a late sign that needs rapid correction.

Feel for pulses, both peripheral and central, assessing for rate, quality, regularity and equality. Treatment and monitoring are covered in detail in Chapters 7 and 8 but should be directed towards haemorrhage control and restoration of tissue perfusion. You must remember that no amount of fluid replacement will be of use in the face of on going severe haemorrhage. Immediate surgery to control haemorrhage may be required at this stage as the only effective form of resuscitation. More frequently, urgent, but non-immediate, surgery will be needed to stop lesser degrees of continued haemorrhage.

Shocked patients fall into three categories:
- the obviously exsanguinating patient who needs immediate definitive treatment (usually surgery) to save their life
- the unstable patient who needs rapid resuscitation and repeated re-assessment over a short period while the cause is identified and treated. They may appear to respond transiently to aggressive fluid resuscitation. Urgent definitive treatment is essential
- the patient with a relatively minor problem who responds rapidly and adequately to a fluid challenge and who remains stable on re-assessment.

Re-assessment (which occurs continuously in the initial stages) simply determines whether the patient is responding to treatment or not. Clearly, if there is no response (or only a transient or inadequate response), different treatment is needed immediately. Patients requiring large and on going volumes of infusion are not stable, even if you can maintain reasonable vital signs.

The fluid challenge can be repeated and colloid solutions can be used provided you are aware of their different distribution and side effects (see Chapter 7, Shock). Only occasionally is it necessary to give uncross-matched blood as type-specific blood is relatively safe and can be obtained within 10–20 minutes. Blood is presently the best resuscitation fluid for the bleeding patient who has cardiovascular instability and who requires, as a guide, more than 1500–2000 ml of resuscitation fluid.

Avoid 'blindly' continuing to transfuse the patient who, in reality, needs surgery. Bleeding patients who need immediate surgery are encountered on the ward at least as frequently as in the emergency room – patients with postoperative bleeding or recurrent bleeding from a peptic ulcer who are pale and shocked are typical examples. As you resuscitate these patients, you should be calling for senior help, cross-matching 8 units of blood and alerting theatre, the anaesthetist and the porters. Shocked or hypotensive patients who are not bleeding are also seen regularly – again, do not continue to 'blindly' fill up a patient with litres of fluid without a clear diagnosis, a clear plan or senior review (preferably all three!). Most surgeons have failed to respond adequately to continuing haemorrhage at some point during their career – so re-assess and reconsider and do not leave a patient with inadequate perfusion without further adequate treatment.

### PRACTICE POINT

*Most unwell surgical patients benefit from administration of oxygen and fluids while further assessment is undertaken.*

*Re-assess as resuscitation proceeds – it often takes more than one assessment to decide on all aspects of the problem.*

## D – DYSFUNCTION OF THE CVP

In the initial assessment, a rapid determination of neurological status is performed by examining the pupils and by using the AVPU system:

- A – Alert
- V – responds to Verbal stimulus
- P – responds only to Pain
- U – Unresponsive to any stimulus.

Remember that the surgical patient may have alteration of conscious level due to causes other than a primary brain injury. Hypoxia with or without hypercarbia and cerebral underperfusion due to shock should have already been detected. Recent administration of sedatives, analgesics or anaesthetic drugs may be responsible. Hypoglycaemia is a common and sometimes overlooked cause that you should look for and treat. If you have thought of all these and the patient is still not fully conscious, re-assess and review the ABCs: you might have missed something.

## E – EXPOSURE

In order to make accurate diagnoses and allow access to the patient for therapeutic manoeuvres, it is essential that the patient is adequately exposed. Be aware that this allows the patient to become cold and exposes patients to the view of others so respect their dignity at all times.

## END OF IMMEDIATE MANAGEMENT

By the end of the phase of immediate assessment and management, the patient should be showing signs of improvement and progressing out of immediate danger. You will very likely have called for help and the patient may have been to theatre or moved to intensive care before this point is reached.

By this stage, the patient should be receiving oxygen and intravenous fluids. If not done already, attach a pulse oximeter, check the blood pressure and confirm that the saturation ($SaO_2$) is above 94%. Arrange pressing investigations not already requested that are targeted and integral to the immediate assessment (perhaps gases, chest X-ray or ECG), insert a urinary catheter (if appropriate) and, if necessary, alert senior colleagues (if you have not already done so). Before you start the next phase, quickly re-assess the ABCs.

### PRACTICE POINT

*If, at any time during the immediate assessment, the patient's condition deteriorates, you must re-assess the ABCs.*

Having initiated resuscitative manoeuvres, it will often take a few minutes for their effects to be apparent. Vital signs may not yet be normal but, provided the patient's condition is improving, you should use the time to continue with the next stage of assessment in order to determine the underlying cause of deterioration. Patients differ (as do their problems); this system is an outline, not an immutable series of commands. However, if the patient is not improving, then re-assess swiftly, get help and arrange for further immediate treatment as appropriate.

## ASSESSMENT OF THE 'STABLE' SURGICAL PATIENT

In many surgical patients, particularly during ward rounds, the vital signs will be normal. Often this can be determined simply by looking at the patient, by asking how they are and asking the nurse how the patient is doing. This essentially social introduction not only establishes rapport and relieves anxiety but also gives information regarding the ABCs, as it does with an acutely ill patient. However, always ask yourself whether the ABCs are normal; if doubt exists, a detailed immediate assessment should be performed. Using the system in this way can avoid simple errors, particularly when you are tired or stressed; it will also let you get to this point in a few seconds with stable patients.

## FULL PATIENT ASSESSMENT

Now that the patient has been immediately stabilised, as necessary, the aim is to gather information from a variety of sources, which will lead to a diagnosis of current or potential problems and, hence, to a plan of action. Your immediate management manoeuvres are not an end in themselves – they simply buy time to solve the underlying problems. The full assessment incorporates a review of the charts and available results plus a full history and examination.

### CHART REVIEWS

Inspection of the observation and fluid charts, preferably at the end of the bed, together with discussion with nursing and other junior medical staff, may bring to light any recent or outstanding

problems. It also allows a more focused clinical assessment to be carried out. Charts, particularly those in HDU or ICU, may appear to carry an overwhelming amount of data but this too can be handled by breaking the chart into sections and systematically noting both absolute values and trends (Table 2.1).

It is not possible to give a comprehensive account of management for every potential scenario but you should consider both general and specific aspects of care. For example, general care includes cardiorespiratory function and fluid balance; alternatively, following liver surgery, one might look specifically for production or drainage of bile, liver function tests, albumin, glucose and clotting factor levels.

### TABLE 2.1

**LOGICAL APPROACH TO HDU CHARTS**

R **Respiratory**
Respiratory rate
Inspired oxygen concentration ($FiO_2$)
Oxygen saturation ($SaO_2$)

C **Circulation**
Heart rate and rhythm
Blood pressure
Urinary output
Fluid balance
Intravenous lines
Central venous pressure
Cardiac output measurements

S **Surgical**
Special requirements of this operation
Temperature
Drainages (nature and volume)

Check the drug chart to see what new drugs have been given and which of the patient's usual drugs might have been forgotten: either may be influencing the current clinical findings.

## HISTORY AND SYSTEMATIC EXAMINATION

The history of the patient's present illness and subsequent treatment is just as important in critical illness as in the rest of clinical practice. However, the impact of co-morbid conditions is almost as great and these are overlooked or underestimated at considerable peril. The patient, the case notes, nursing and junior medical staff are the main sources of these types of information and the appropriate source will vary from case to case, depending on your prior knowledge of the patient. On occasion, family and other professional staff can also supply useful information.

The patient is then examined fully with particular attention being paid to vital systems, the systems or regions involved by surgery or underlying disease and to potential problems already highlighted. This should follow the standard format, beginning with the hands, and include neck, chest, abdomen and limbs. Wounds or stomas may also require examination. The importance of repeated clinical examination is often underestimated by inexperienced staff, particularly when it comes to diagnosing incipient problems in silent areas; for example, early signs of atelectasis are much more likely to be detected clinically than radiologically. Equally, we all fail to pick up on subtle signs. Repeated examination, perhaps after 15 minutes, helps to prevent this (Case Scenario 2.1).

## CASE SCENARIO 2.1

You are on the orthopaedic ward at 3 a.m. with a trauma case when you are asked to see a 48-year-old male patient who is tachycardic (HR 110), 12 h after a spinal cord decompression. The main ward lights are not on, the patient is distressed and in pain and the foundation year doctor has just started a 500ml bolus fluid challenge and prescribed more analgesia. Blood pressure is 105/75. You think the patient is a little cool peripherally but are not unduly concerned. You have a cup of coffee and then review the patient again. You realise that, despite 500 ml of saline, his perfusion is worse, he is oliguric and has a distended abdomen. It is now clear to you that the patient may well have continuing surgical bleeding and that more intensive resuscitation and consideration of urgent re-operation is required.

### LEARNING POINT
- Re-assessment after a short period of time or following a simple intervention often helps clarify the diagnosis.

## REVIEW OF AVAILABLE RESULTS

Available investigation results should now be reviewed (Table 2.2). With emergencies, a great deal of useful data may be available from previous routine blood results microbiology samples or recent imaging requests, so do not overlook this source of information. On routine ward rounds it can be better to wait at the end of the bed for missing results than to resolve to 'see them later' – experience suggests that these tasks slip the memory in the busy routine. Work out a schedule with your junior colleagues that maximises the availability of recent results for your main business ward rounds, including an up-to-date file of all patients on your ward.

### TABLE 2.2

#### REVIEW AVAILABLE RESULTS

- Biochemistry profile
  - ABG's
  - Glucose level
- Haematology
  - Blood count
  - Clotting
  - Cross-matched blood available
- Microbiology
- Radiology
  - Review reports or examine films
- ECG
- Return to charts and review any necessary points

## DECIDE AND PLAN – STABLE OR UNSTABLE?

Once you have assessed the patient and the available information, you need to make a decision – is the patient stable or unstable? Patients about whom you are unsure should be managed as if unstable. Also, you should be very cautious about assigning patients who have been unstable, but who have just responded to treatment, to the stable group too quickly. Clearly, there are degrees of instability but training yourself to make this simple decision is important as it will focus your mind on to one of two very different subsequent approaches.

### STABLE PATIENTS – DAILY PLAN

Stable patients have normal signs and are progressing as expected. This will apply to most patients seen on the daily ward round and, consequently, they will not need the aggressive 'immediate management' for unstable patients. It is your duty to formulate a management plan. On the ward this will be daily (Table 2.3); however, in HDU, 12-hourly or more frequent assessment and planning will be needed.

Ensure that necessary therapeutic drugs, including analgesia, are prescribed. Modify these as the patient recovers. Check that appropriate prophylaxis, particularly against venous thrombo-embolism, is prescribed. Verify that routine medications are being given (if necessary by an alternative route) and consider what implications the co-morbid condition or its treatment might have for present management or prognosis.

Remember also to speak to the patient, to encourage and reassure them. Sum up your plan with clear instructions for your nursing colleagues and junior staff and make or supervise an entry in the notes.

## PRACTICE POINT

*Plan and sum up, communicate and document.*

## TABLE 2.3

### DAILY PLAN

- Investigations
  - Blood tests and X-rays, specialist opinions
- Removal of drains/tubes
- Oral intake
- Fluid balance and prescription
- Nutrition
  - Requirement
  - Route
  - Is it being given?
- Physiotherapy
  - Chest and mobility
- Drugs and analgesia
  - Therapeutic (*e.g.* antibiotics, analgesia)
  - Preventative (*e.g.* subcutaneous heparin)
  - Routine (*e.g.* cardiac)
- Move to lower level of care

## UNSTABLE PATIENTS

If progress is not satisfactory, further investigation or definitive treatment will be needed. If a cause is already evident from your evaluation, treatment can be planned directly. Inform your senior and consider whether a higher level of care is needed.

When the patient is unstable or you are unsure:
- review priorities
- is resuscitation required before you begin investigations (often the case)?
- does it need to be continued simultaneously with proposed investigations (usually the case)?
- how will you achieve that?
- begin any treatment or support that is obviously necessary at once
- does the patient need a higher level of care?

## SPECIFIC TARGETED INVESTIGATIONS

These are carried out as necessary to find out why the patient is unstable and to let you or others do something about it subsequently. These range from the simple to the very complex. Usually, simple blood tests will have already been sent off during the immediate management phase but now is the time to check. Likewise, chest radiographs, ECGs and various cultures may have already been done or may be needed now.

The safest way to accomplish more complex and specific investigations will differ between patients depending on the test required, the degree of urgency and how sick the patient is. Remember the radiology department is an unsafe place for sick patients unless they have adequate critical care support from medical and nursing staff. The ideal test may have to be foregone in some circumstances or it may be better to transfer the patient to ICU for full support before a planned transfer to the radiology department. Specialist opinions (*e.g.* cardiology, anaesthesia, intensive care) may be required. If you reach an impasse, either of a diagnostic or organisational nature, involve your senior colleagues. If you are unsure at this stage, ask for help! However, do not give up on a necessary investigation or treatment just because it is difficult to arrange, an awkward time or beyond your expertise. Unstable patients seldom improve spontaneously between 4–8 a.m. (Case Scenario 2.2).

## CASE SCENARIO 2.2

An elderly patient with known mild heart failure underwent endoscopy and diathermy of a bleeding duodenal ulcer at 8 p.m. He became steadily oliguric from 11 p.m. and had two cautious fluid challenges from the junior ward doctor. You are asked to see him at 3.35 a.m. and note he is not well perfused and mildly dyspnoeic. You give a further 350 ml saline over 45 minutes without any change in the patient's condition. You are unsure what fluids are required and feel a central line is needed. You are aware this needs to be performed by an anaesthetist but there is only a consultant on call after midnight. You elect to continue with maintenance fluids until the 8 a.m. ward round so as not to bother the consultant overnight. By then, the patient is anuric and in established renal failure.

### LEARNING POINTS

- Patients do not improve magically between 4 a.m. and the 8 a.m. ward round!
- Unstable patients require diagnosis and definitive treatment without undue delay
- Involve senior staff if you do not have the particular skills to deal with a given problem.

Be careful to maintain momentum – on busy wards, multiple small delays at each stage can add up to a lengthy delay in treating the underlying cause, which can result in your previous resuscitation being in vain.

Investigations may take some time, during which you must ask yourself repeatedly:

- is the present level of physiological support optimal?
- are we reaching a diagnosis and a definite plan of action?
- are we doing so quickly enough?

If not, a change of plan is needed!

When you have attended a patient, you must record the event in the case notes (Table 2.4). This serves several functions – writing your assessment helps clarify your thoughts, your note tells other staff what happened and lets them gauge the response, you can define clear criteria for further interventions and the note can be of medicolegal importance.

| TABLE 2.4 |
|---|

WRITING YOUR NOTES

- Name in capitals, date and time, pager number
- Assessment
- Brief summary of past and present events
  Present clinical features
  Response to any treatment already given
  (*e.g.* by foundation year doctor)
- Differential diagnosis
- Actions
  Resuscitation performed (ABC)
  Investigations and opinions
  Treatment
- Communications to relatives, staff, seniors, etc.
- Review
  By you
  By others
- Parameters for change

## DEFINITIVE TREATMENT

The underlying aim of critical care practice is to begin definitive treatment of continuing pathology or complications as quickly as possible. All the above steps simply keep the patient alive long enough to get this far; however, unless you treat the real problem adequately, the patient will deteriorate again and may die. Once the need for intervention is clear to all, the situation may be irretrievable so speed is of the essence throughout.

Treatment may be medical, surgical or radiological or all three: co-ordination is important. When the patient is a surgical one, you will need to play a leading role in co-ordinating efforts. Consider where non-operative treatment should best be carried out, by whom and what support will be necessary. If the patient is transferred, especially to an area unfamiliar with surgical patients (*e.g.* coronary care unit), detailed instructions will need to be written in the case notes and frequent review will be necessary to ensure that other surgical aspects of care continue to be delivered even though the staff are unfamiliar with them.

## RE-ASSESSMENT

Finally, once any treatment has been instituted, whether simple fluid therapy or a complex surgical operation, you must re-assess the patient to ensure that they have responded to the treatment. The necessary time frame for doing this will depend on the urgency of the case.

If they have not responded adequately, then you need to look all the harder for a different cause to treat. Re-assessment is the final step – and, if necessary, the first step in repeating the whole process.

## SUMMARY

This system will let you assess all your patients in a similar way. It is the system that many senior surgeons and intensivists have used subconsciously for a long time, just in written form. With practice, the use of a system will let you assess patients without overlooking simple and potentially disastrous things and it will serve as a framework whereby you can apply your theoretical knowledge to clinical problems.

- using a structured system to assess critically ill patients reduces serious omissions
- identify those in need of immediate life-saving resuscitation – assess and treat them simultaneously
- reach a diagnosis that accounts for clinical deterioration
- formulate and institute a plan of definitive treatment
- investigations should be selective and carried out in a safe environment
- repeated clinical assessment is the cornerstone of good practice – it identifies things missed first time around and tells you whether the patient is getting better
- inform and involve your senior colleagues at an early stage
- consider the level of care necessary at each stage
- communicate and document at all times.

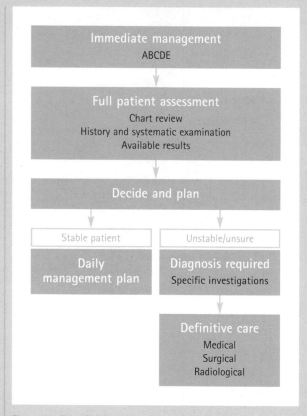

Figure 2.1 The CCrISP system of assessment.

# 3

Airway and
tracheostomy
management

This chapter will help you to:

- understand the basic principles of airway management
- recognise the indications for tracheostomies in critically ill patients and the indications for their removal
- understand how to deal with some common complications of tracheostomies.

## AIRWAY MANAGEMENT

The commonesty reason for admission to an ICU is to provide airway and ventilatory care to critically ill patients who are unable to maintain their own airway and normal respiratory functions. The early recognition of an airway or ventilatory problem together with early appropriate treatment will often prevent further deterioration and is the basis of effective resuscitation. Many more patients on surgical wards exhibit signs of respiratory compromise and their effective management is a sizeable and important part of surgical critical care.

As outlined in Chapter 2, you should look specifically for an airway problem when assessing every patient. Often, the patient will respond verbally but, if not, you should suspect airway compromise in any obtunded patient. Alteration in the level of consciousness, for whatever reason, will result in loss of airway control, decreased or loss of protective gag and/or laryngeal reflexes and increased risk of aspiration of gastric contents into the lungs.

Problems with the airway are generally quite intimidating for surgical trainees: an unconscious patient with no airway must be resuscitated quickly to prevent hypoxic brain damage. Remember the ABC approach of the CCrISP algorithm also applies in cases of apparent airway problems. You can review how airway management fits into this system in Chapter 2.

The patient with airway and/or breathing difficulties may be easily recognised if they are:
- dyspnoeic, tachypnoeic or apnoeic
- unable to speak in complete sentences
- using accessory muscles of respiration
- centrally cyanosed
- sweaty and tachycardic
- showing a decreased level of consciousness or becoming agitated and difficult to control.

There are two golden rules to airway management: (i) always give oxygen in the highest concentration possible; and (ii) use simple methods first.

## TECHNIQUES OF AIRWAY CONTROL

If the patient is still breathing, use high flow oxygen masks (*e.g.* Hudson mask) with a reservoir bag (Fig. 3.1). During resuscitation, you should not worry about the possibility of depressing ventilation by giving high concentrations of oxygen to a patient who normally requires a hypoxic drive to produce adequate ventilation. Hypoxia kills people quicker than loss of respiratory drive and the condition is rarely seen in surgical patients.

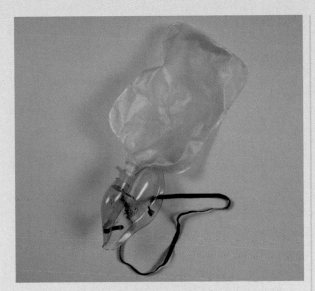

Figure 3.1 **High flow oxygen mask with reservoir bag.**

Apply a pulse oximeter to allow you to assess that oxygen administration is improving the patient's saturations. Once the patient has stabilised, the oxygen concentration can be decreased to maintain adequate saturations: pulse oximetry can guide this. Remember that pulse oximetry does not indicate hypercapnia.

## ESCALATING AIRWAY SUPPORT

In increasing measure, airway support can be achieved by: (i) chin lift/jaw thrust; (ii) suction; (iii) oral Guedel airway or nasopharyngeal airway if gag reflex present; (iv) laryngeal mask or endotracheal tube; and (v) surgical airway.

Basic manoeuvres without airway adjuncts are often sufficient to improve gas exchange through a compromised airway. If not, an oral Guedel airway should be inserted (Fig. 3.2). This is sized from the angle of the mandible to the mouth, and inserted upside down and rotated as it is inserted.

Have suction on hand at all times. A nasopharyngeal airway may be inserted if the patient has a gag reflex.

In situations of airway compromise, call for help early. In particular, seek anaesthetic/critical care help at any point if you are unable to cope or think you may reach the limits of your competency. Patients who are semiconscious and unable to tolerate an oral airway will not tolerate endotracheal intubation or laryngeal mask insertion without additional sedation and so you must seek additional help to secure the airway. If the patient is apnoeic or has very shallow respiration then ventilation using a bag/valve /mask system is required (Fig. 3.3). This can usually maintain the patient until an anaesthetist arrives. With appropriate training, attempting to insert a laryngeal mask airway can often be simpler, quicker and easier than attempting intubation. If you do decide to attempt intubation, you should keep in mind the risk of regurgitation and aspiration of stomach contents and apply cricoid pressure prior to laryngoscopy. Neither technique should be attempted by the inexperienced trainee - help must be sought!

If you try to intubate the patient and fail, or if you are unable to ventilate the patient manually or with a laryngeal mask airway, then you are committed to performing a surgical airway by either needle or surgical cricothyroidotomy in order to ensure life-saving oxygenation and ventilation. The techniques of airway management are covered in the Advanced Trauma Life Support® (ATLS®) course and will not be covered in further detail in the CCrISP course.

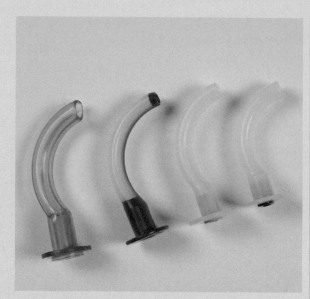
Figure 3.2 Geudel airway.

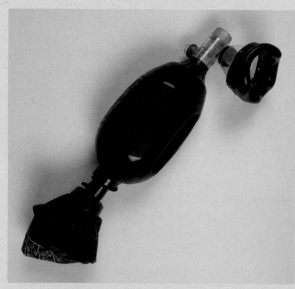
Figure 3.3 Bag/valve/mask system.

## TRACHEOSTOMY

Tracheostomy is commonly performed in patients in the ICU, mostly using variations of the Seldinger guidewire technique as a planned bedside procedure. There is currently no evidence that one technique is superior to the other, and often the chosen technique will depend as much on local practice as patient factors. Indications for tracheostomy are listed in Table 3.1.

| TABLE 3.1 |
| --- |
| **INDICATIONS FOR TRACHEOSTOMY IN CRITICALLY ILL PATIENTS**<br>– Weaning from mechanical ventilation<br>– Bronchial toilet (excessive secretions, poor cough)<br>– Protect the airway (*e.g.* following CVA)<br>– Maintain the airway (*e.g.* upper airway obstruction) |

Tracheostomies are increasingly being performed early in a patient's stay on the ICU and, in some hospitals, patients with tracheostomies are being managed on non-ENT wards. It is, therefore, important for surgeons to be aware of, prevent and deal with the common complications of tracheostomy.

### TYPES OF TRACHEOSTOMY

Tracheostomy tubes can vary depending on the needs of the patient and the problems the tracheostomy is intended to overcome. They are constructed from either a form of plastic or metal. Documentation of the type of tube and size should be in the patient's notes and this should always be checked where possible. Other features of tracheostomy tubes are listed in Table 3.2 and illustrated in Fig. 3.4.

## TABLE 3.2

### FEATURES OF TRACHEOSTOMY TUBES

| Tracheostomy feature | Further information |
|---|---|
| Cuffed versus uncuffed | Cuffed tubes are required for mechanical ventilatory support but do not allow speech |
| Single lumen versus inner cannula | Inner cannula can be removed for cleaning without loss of the tracheostomy as the outer tube remains in place. Safer long term |
| Fixed versus adjustable flange | Adjustable flange tubes can be used to overcome short-term anatomical problems such as swollen neck but are not suitable for longer term use |
| Fenestrated versus non-fenestrated | Fenestrations allow patients to talk with a tracheostomy tube *in situ*. Not used in ventilated patients |

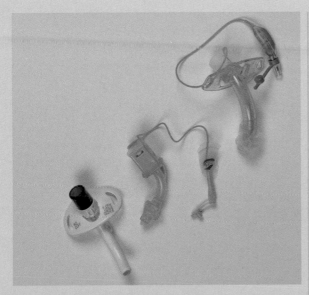

Figure 3.4 Selection of tracheostomy tubes.

Information on tube size should be located on the flange; unfortunately, there is no uniformity of tracheostomy tube size with regard to length and dimensions so this needs to be checked for each type of tube. As a general rule, most adult females can accommodate a tube with an outer diameter of 10 mm, while for most men a tube with an outer diameter of 11 mm is suitable. Selecting appropriate tube size is important to maximise the internal tube dimensions and reduce the work of breathing through the tube. However, an over-sized tube can cause pressure necrosis and damage the tracheal mucosa. A tracheostomy tube that is too small will need over-inflation of the cuff to prevent accidental displacement.

## WARD MANAGEMENT OF PATIENTS WITH A TRACHEOSTOMY

Management of tracheostomies on the ward is usually straightforward, provided simple principles are followed:

- humidification and regular suction are essential: it is often lack of basic toileting of the airway that leads to tracheostomy blockage
- apply the CCrISP algorithm when asked to deal with a tracheostomy problem or review the continuing need for one
- determine when the procedure was performed and what type of tracheostomy the patient received. Tubes should not be changed within 3 days of a surgical procedure, and ideally not within 7-10 days of a percutaneous procedure, to ensure that the track has formed properly
- on the wards, single lumen tubes are generally unfavourable due to the risk of blockage. These should be replaced with a tracheostomy with a removable inner tube to facilitate cleaning as soon as it is safe to do so.

### PRACTICE POINT

*Tracheostomy tubes should only be changed by staff who have the necessary competencies. If you have not had relevant training you will not have competency in this area and should not plan to undertake the procedure unsupervised.*

## COMPLICATIONS OF TRACHEOSTOMY

The commonest major complications are blockage, displacement and haemorrhage.

*Blockage or displacement*

A blocked or displaced tracheostomy tube generally presents with respiratory compromise. Always use the CCrISP algorithm: remember there may be other cardiorespiratory reasons for breathing difficulties, which may be missed without a systematic approach. A partially displaced tracheostomy tube is just as dangerous as a blocked or completely removed tube. The key factor to determine is if the airway is patent.

If the tube is displaced, the patient may be breathing through their nose or mouth. It will usually be safer to remove a partly dislodged tube. The patient can be given oxygen via facemask and monitored in the short term with pulse oximetry.

If there are problems once the tracheostomy has been removed, you should not try to replace it. Maintain the airway by other methods until experienced help arrives.

If you bag/mask ventilate a patient after removal of the tracheostomy tube, air will escape from the stoma and you will need an assistant to occlude the stoma by hand and an occlusive dressing to reduce the leak.

If the tube is partially blocked, the patient may still be able to breathe through it with difficulty:

- encourage the patient to cough as this may dislodge any blockage
- pass a suction catheter down the tube
- oxygen should be given via the tracheostomy and also via a facemask
- if the tube has an inner cannula, this should be removed and changed

- if the tube has a single lumen tube and a suction catheter can be passed, it must be partially patent: the patient can be monitored and given oxygen until the arrival of expert help
- if the patient cannot breathe spontaneously via the stoma, establish an airway by other means. Call for help at this point if you have not already done so!

*Haemorrhage*
Tracheostomy site bleeding on the ward may occur because of erosion of blood vessels in and around the stoma site. Bleeding may settle with conservative management. However, if it results from erosion of a major artery in the root of the neck, the bleeding will be massive and is a life-threatening emergency. This should be managed as follows:
- try not to panic, call for help (anaesthetic and surgical) and adopt the CCrISP algorithm
- reassure the patient
- inspect the stoma site for any obvious bleeding point and apply manual pressure
- if still bleeding, infiltrate any obvious bleeding point with dilute adrenaline (1:80,000 to 1:200,000)
- if no obvious bleeding point, infiltrate the stoma margins generally
- check full blood count and a coagulation screen. Correct any abnormalities and ensure blood for transfusion is available
- bleeding may be temporarily stemmed by applying pressure to the root of the neck in the sternal notch or by inflating the cuff slowly, taking care not to burst it. Depending on the type and size of the tube, this may need a volume of 10–35 ml

- call for senior surgical help if you have not already done so as the patient needs surgical exploration, preferably by an ENT or maxillofacial surgeon.

## TRACHEOSTOMY TUBE REMOVAL
Reviewing the continuing need for a tracheostomy should be part of the daily patient plan. It is important to remove a tracheostomy as soon as it is no longer required and the initial indication for its presence has passed. If the patient can cough, expectorate, phonate and protect the airway with the cuff deflated, and is maintaining good oxygen saturations on minimal oxygen concentrations, the prospects for decannulation are good. The best time for decannulation is usually in the morning as the patient has rested overnight and their condition can be observed during the remainder of the day. Some hospitals are able to provide assessments from speech and language therapy as to swallowing and laryngeal competence but this is not universal. The use of specialised tracheostomy tubes requires input from your ENT or ICU colleagues.

If you do not know how to replace/change a tube, always ask for help before you start. Depending on the hospital, this may be obtained from a critical care out-reach team, anaesthesia, physiotherapy or other staff.

As a general rule, the following steps are necessary:
- ensure that the appropriate equipment is available (Table 3.3)
- monitor the patient with pulse oximetry as a minimum. Be aware that suctioning can cause bradycardia
- ensure the patient is receiving supplemental oxygen via the tracheostomy mask

- inform the patient about the procedure and ensure he or she understands
- position the patient so that he or she is comfortable with the neck slightly extended if possible
- suction the tube using an endobronchial suction catheter
- deflate cuff after ensuring patient's pharynx is empty with oral suctioning
- remove the tube
- after decannulation, dress and occlude the stoma with sterile gauze covered with an occlusive tape dressing
- give the patient supplemental oxygen via a facemask or nasal cannulae
- observe the patient for signs of respiratory distress.

## TABLE 3.3

### EQUIPMENT FOR REMOVAL OF A TRACHEOSTOMY TUBE

- Operational suction unit with suction tubing attached and Yankaeur sucker
- Endobronchial suction catheters
- Gloves, aprons and eye protection
- Spare tracheostomy tubes of the same type as inserted: one the same size and one a size smaller
- Tracheal dilator forceps
- Self-inflating reservoir bag and tubing
- Catheter mount
- Tracheostomy tube holder and dressing
- 10 ml syringe (if tube cuffed)
- Resuscitation equipment

Risks of tracheostomy removal include airway obstruction, aspiration, ventilatory failure, sputum retention and difficulty with oral re-intubation if required.

### SUMMARY

- there are two golden rules to airway management in surgical patients – always give oxygen in the highest concentration possible and use simple methods for airway control first
- seek anaesthetic/critical care help at any point if you are unable to cope or think you may reach the limits of your competency
- common complications of tracheostomy in ward patients are accidental displacement, blockage and haemorrhage
- surgeons need to be aware of and be able to deal with these complications and how to avoid them by appropriate ward-based management. Be aware of when and who to call for additional expert help.

### FURTHER READING

Standards for the care of adult patients with a temporary tracheostomy. Intensive Care Society, July 2008. Available at <http://www.ics.ac.uk>.

*Advanced Trauma Life Support for Doctors. ATLS® Student Course Manual.* 8th edn. Chicago, IL: American College of Surgeons; 2008.

# 4

Respiratory
compromise in
the surgical patient

**OBJECTIVES**

This chapter will help you to:

- understand the importance of respiratory failure and its prevention
- recognise the patient with respiratory failure and the need for support
- provide a management approach to respiratory failure
- be familiar with common methods of respiratory support
- understand the basic concepts of mechanical ventilation.

## INTRODUCTION

Respiratory failure is an acute or chronic failure of oxygenation, manifesting as a $PaO_2$ of less than 8 kPa, due to inadequate pulmonary gas exchange. A $PaO_2$ of 8 kPa is the point on the oxygen dissociation curve when rapid desaturation occurs if there is any further fall in $PaO_2$ (Fig. 4.1). Respiratory failure represents the commonest cause of a decreased level of consciousness in general surgical patients and is classified depending on the $CO_2$ level:

- *Type I failure* – failed oxygen uptake leads to hypoxia ($PaO_2$ of less than 8 kPa: normal range, 10.6–13.3 kPa) but normal or reduced $PaCO_2$ (normal range, 4.7–6.0 kPa)
- *Type II failure* – failed oxygen uptake and carbon dioxide removal leads to hypoxia and hypercarbia ($PaCO_2$ of greater than 6.7 kPa).

There are a number of common causes of respiratory failure in the surgical patient, which can be classified into three broad groups:

- *Acute fall in functional residual capacity without pulmonary vascular dysfunction* – includes central or myoneural disorders, failure of chest mechanics after trauma or other processes that render the lungs stiff and non-compliant. Acute postoperative atelectasis, sputum retention, pneumonia or depression of respiration by analgesic, sedative or neuromuscular blocking drugs fall into this category. Frailty and malnutrition contribute
- *Acute fall in FRC with pulmonary vascular dysfunction* – includes left ventricular failure, fluid overload, pulmonary hypertension, pulmonary embolism, neurogenic pulmonary oedema or ARDS
- *Airflow obstruction* – including increased lung volume states such as chronic obstructive pulmonary disease, asthma or other airflow obstruction.

Factors that increase the risk of respiratory problems include:

- history of pre-existing respiratory disease, such as asthma, COPD and obstructive sleep apnoea
- smoking
- thoracic surgery
- upper abdominal surgery
- obesity
- elderly.

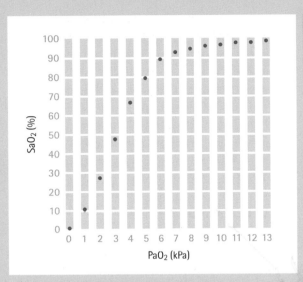

Figure 4.1 The oxygen haemoglobin dissociation curve. Below a $PaO_2$ of 8 kPa the slope drops away steeply. Keep the saturation > 94% to ensure the $PaO_2$ is above 8 kPa!

## IMMEDIATE ASSESSMENT AND MANAGEMENT

Although the precise definition of respiratory failure is based on ABG criteria, the initial assessment and management approach should follow the systematic approach of the CCrISP algorithm.

Remember the ABCs. An unconscious patient with no airway must be resuscitated quickly to prevent hypoxic brain damage. Review airway management in Chapters 2 and 3.

Patients with respiratory failure may be easily recognised if they are:

● dypnoeic, tachypnoeic or apnoeic
● unable to speak in complete sentences
● using accessory muscles of respiration
● centrally cyanosed
● sweating and tachycardic, and/or
● showing a decreased level of consciousness.

Aim to oxygenate the patient using high flow oxygen masks of suitable oxygen delivery percentages if the patient is still breathing. Remember, during resuscitation, you should not worry about the possibility of depressing ventilation by giving high concentrations of oxygen to a patient with chronic pulmonary disease who normally requires a hypoxic drive to produce adequate ventilation having become habituated to a high level of arterial carbon dioxide. If the patient needs oxygen that badly you should give it!

Apply a pulse oximeter. Once the patient has stabilised, the rule is to give the minimum added oxygen to achieve the best oxygenation.

## PULSE OXIMETRY

Pulse oximetry has become a central tool in the monitoring of critically ill surgical patients. It represents a continuous method of monitoring oxygen saturations, not absolute oxygen levels or ventilation.

Understanding the mechanism will make you aware of the limitations. Pulse oximetry works by combining two principles based on light transmission and reception through the tissue. First, the probe detects pulsatile flow plethysmographically. Second, it differentiates between oxygenated and reduced haemoglobin by their differing light absorption. Signal processing produces a display of heart rate and arterial oxygen saturation ($SaO_2$).

Remember that the saturation does not equate to the partial pressure (which is responsible for gas exchange) – the oxygen dissociation curve in Fig. 4.1 links these parameters. Note that $SaO_2$ of 94% often equates with a $PaO_2$ of approximately 8 kPa so it is advisable to aim to keep the $SaO_2$ above 94% and to set the alarms accordingly. There is a delay of around 20 seconds between actual and displayed values.

The pulse oximeter does not detect hypercarbia or acidosis – these require blood gas analysis.

The pulse oximeter is fooled by carboxyhaemoglobin into giving an erroneously high reading. Other factors that impede accurate pulse oximetry include:

- movement: shivering, rigors, tremor, agitation
- peripheral vasoconstriction – shock, hypothermia
- dirty skin/pigmentation including jaundice/ nail varnish
- cardiac arrhythmias
- profound anaemia
- diathermy
- bright lights
- when the $SaO_2$ is lower than 70%.

## FULL PATIENT ASSESSMENT

### CHART REVIEW
Chart examination may reveal changes in respiratory rate, temperature, pulse rate, blood pressure, change in colour or amount of sputum produced, change in level of consciousness or a fall in oxygen saturation or deterioration in ABG if previously recorded. Fluid balance charts should be examined for signs of fluid overload. A deteriorating trend in any of these physiological variables is an essential diagnostic tool and accurate charting cannot be over emphasised.

### HISTORY AND SYSTEMATIC EXAMINATION
You should rapidly review the patient's history in an effort to determine the likely source of

respiratory difficulty. The patient may be a known asthmatic, chronic bronchitic or may recently have received a large dose of opiates. If this information is obtainable from the nurses, you can be simultaneously examining the patient. The examination should initially be clinical, based on simple 'Look, Listen and Feel' techniques described in the assessment chapter and aimed at detecting the physiological changes of developing respiratory failure.

### AVAILABLE RESULTS
*Full blood count:* correction of anaemia will help to improve oxygen delivery to the tissues if the haemoglobin is less than 10 g/dl. Over-transfusion, conversely, brings the risk of fluid overload and increased blood viscosity. An elevated white cell count may indicate concurrent infection that may be pneumonic in origin.

The *urea and electrolytes* may give some indication of fluid and renal status.

*ABG sampling* is the single most useful blood test in relation to respiratory failure. You should be familiar with the practical skill of sampling and the interpretation of these results. The interpretation of ABGs is outlined in Chapter 5. Remember to treat the patient as a whole and not to act only on the blood gases in isolation from the clinical findings.

The *ECG* will provide information regarding the presence or absence of myocardial ischaemia, rhythm and rate, abnormalities of which may be responsible for the onset or worsening of respiratory failure. Cardiac and respiratory physiological variables are inseparable when it comes to assessment and treatment of respiratory failure, and further investigations of cardiac function such as echocardiography or cardiac output or index estimations may be appropriate at a higher level of care.

The *plain chest X-ray* remains a valuable diagnostic tool but transfer of the unstable patient to the radiology department is dangerous and should not delay treatment. Radiographic changes often lag behind the clinical changes and it is important to treat the patient, not the X-ray. Interpretation of chest X-rays must follow a systematic approach as described in Table 4.1.

Pre-operative *lung function tests* (peak expiratory flow rate, vital capacity and $FEV_1$) are useful in predicting the patient at risk although a patient's ability to climb a flight of stairs in one go or to conduct everyday tasks also provides valuable information.

Infection is the most common cause of respiratory failure and samples of sputum and blood for culture should be obtained preferably before commencing antibiotic therapy. If the patient is already on antibiotics, these should be taken before the next dose when antibiotic blood levels are at their lowest. In the intubated patient, sputum samples can be taken by BAL. These give better results since they are uncontaminated by upper airway flora.

## STABLE PATIENT – DAILY MANAGEMENT PLAN

Frequent assessment of all surgical patients, but especially those at high risk, is important. Routinely assess respiratory rate, $SaO_2$ along with oxygen requirements, cyanosis, ability to cough and deep breathe, looking for signs of respiratory distress, sweatiness and tachycardia and formal examination of the chest. If there any concerns, consider the investigations outlined above.

Prescribe humidified oxygen therapy by mask at an appropriate concentration. Monitor clinical signs (especially respiratory rate), oxygen saturation and ABGs. For patients with lower oxygen requirements, nasal cannulae may be used, but remember that oxygen should be administered to patients to keep their $SaO_2$ above 94%. Communicate with nursing staff and ensure that they are aware of the increased frequency of desired observations to be made.

Physiotherapy review should be sought for all patients at risk of, or developing, respiratory problems. Important aspects to be considered are patient positioning, mobilisation, exercises to encourage deep breathing, suction of respiratory secretions using nasopharyngeal airways, techniques such as percussion and use of devices such as incentive spirometry.

Ensure patients are on any routine prescriptions they have for respiratory disease such as inhalers and nebulisers. Consider use of nebulised saline to loosen secretions. If a patient develops wheeze (which can occur in the absence of previous respiratory disease), prescribe nebulised salbutamol and ipratropium. Increasingly, patients are using home NIV or CPAP. Ensure that any patient who uses these devices brings them into hospital with them and that staff who will be looking after them are familiar with their use. Adequate analgesia is important to enable patients to cough and deep breathe. Conversely, over-use of opiates leads to narcotisation, and airway and respiratory compromise.

Set parameters beyond which staff must call for further medical opinion. Commence hourly urine output monitoring if the patient is catheterised and enforce meticulous fluid balance and microbiological surveillance (sputum and blood cultures). Monitor respiratory rate, $SaO_2$, $FiO_2$, BP, heart rate, temperature and AVPU score. For most surgical patients, 4-hourly observations are appropriate but, if you are concerned, increase to hourly. Increasingly, MEWS charts are being used. Abnormalities in observations should be reported to critical care out-reach teams, who will help with liaising with critical care and offer advice.

## CASE SCENARIO 4.1

A 45-year-old man had a laparoscopic gastric bypass 2 days ago. His BMI is 45 kg/$m^2$, and he has a history of obstructive sleep apnoea but has refused home CPAP because of poor tolerance. He has a history of chronic pain problems and normally takes regular paracetamol and oramorph PRN. You are called to see him because his saturations are 90% and he is complaining of pain. He is maintaining an airway and immediate assessment reveals a temperature of 37.3°C, respiratory rate of 24 and $SaO_2$ of 90% on room air. He has not been out of bed since the operation as there is no suitable chair. He also has NIDDM and hypertension. He is cyanosed but well perfused. You review him in detail and find that he has not been receiving his normal analgesia, no oxygen therapy had been given for 6 h and that he had not seen the physiotherapist today. He has poor air entry bilaterally, particularly at the right base. Blood gases now show a mild respiratory acidosis and a $PaCO_2$ just above the upper limit of normal. You prescribe humidified oxygen to maintain his saturation above 95% and start regular nebulised salbutamol as he uses salbutamol as necessary at home. A CXR is requested, which reveals atelectasis at both bases (Fig. 4.2). You arrange for immediate review by the on-call physiotherapist and by the pain team. The physiotherapist obtains a sputum sample for culture but, as this looks clear and as he has a normal white cell count, you elect not to start antibiotics at present. You review him 1 h later, confirm that his improved analgesia has allowed him to increase his air entry and clearance of secretions and thereby, oxygenation. The blood gases have improved. You discuss the case with the nurse and agree the necessary frequency of observations and parameters of saturation, respiratory rate and pain score that would necessitate further urgent medical review. You plan to review in any event at 8 a.m. to discuss with (and feed back to!) the patient's own team.

### LEARNING POINTS
- predict the patients at risk and establish the correct level of care from the outset
- regular nursing observations and medical review – once daily is not enough in some cases
- use preventative techniques including chest physiotherapy, nebulised saline, monitored humidified oxygen, adequate analgesia and sputum culture liberally.

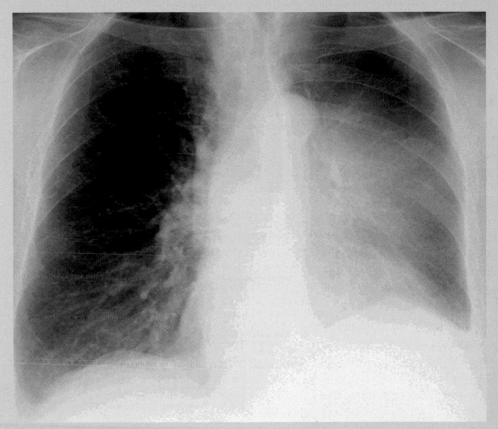

Figure 4.2 CXR confirmed to be a recent film of the patient in Case Scenario 4.1. There is basal shadowing suggestive of marked atelectasis and no other obvious pathology.

## PRACTICE POINT

*The frequency with which early chest problems are encountered cannot be overemphasised, nor can the importance of examining the chest routinely and adopting simple preventive measures liberally.*

## PREVENTING RESPIRATORY DETERIORATION FOLLOWING SURGERY

- identify those at risk
- examine and assess
- chest physiotherapy
- nebulised saline
- humidified oxygen – titrated dose
- adequate analgesia
- sputum culture
- re-assess regularly.

# PRACTICAL SKILL: INTERPRETING CHEST RADIOGRAPHS

## OBJECTIVES

- learn a system for examining chest radiographs in the critically ill
- be aware of the complementary information provided by clinical and radiographic examination.

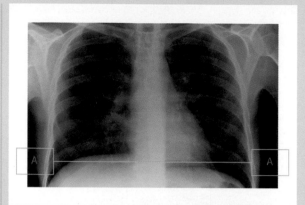

Figure 4.3a Chest x-ray showing the line method of assessment.

The CXR is one of the most frequently ordered investigations in the management of the critically ill. In many cases, abnormal signs will be picked up earlier on clinical examination as radiographic appearances tend to lag behind the clinical findings. The CXR offers valuable confirmatory and complementary diagnostic evidence (or reassurance). The aim here is not to list exhaustively the clinical scenarios and diagnoses where it may be of help, but rather to teach a system of reading a CXR.

Use a routine when looking at chest X-rays: you may miss other pathology if you do not. The most useful chest view for assessing the heart is a straight, erect PA, taken at full inspiration. This type of radiograph is more likely to give a true indication of heart size than the portable AP film which may suggest cardiomegaly. Be aware of which type you are looking at and remember to check name, date and time. Compare with previous films.

Your routine should be:

- note overall shape of the chest and obvious abnormalities
- use a system to assess the CXR fully. One system is the line method (Fig. 4.3a).

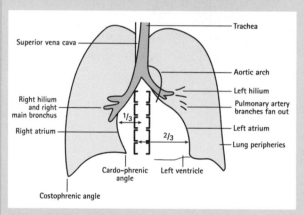

Figure 4.3b Diagrammatic representation of a CXR.

Draw a line across the lower part of the CXR to include the costophrenic angle as shown (A–A). The line passes through the structures to be examined in order:

- *soft tissues*: look for air (surgical emphysema), foreign bodies or disruption of contours
- *bony structures*: use the Collegiate mnemonic RCS'S – comprising ribs, clavicles, scapulae, sternum
- *lung markings*: do they extend to the chest wall? Is there pneumothorax or haemothorax? Trace around the edge of the pleural cavity to

avoid missing a small pneumothorax. Is the volume of parenchyma increased (COAD, lots of ribs visible) or reduced (poor respiratory effort, abdominal distension)
- examine the lung fields for opacities
- double check the costophrenic angles for fluid (erect film?)
- is there air beneath the diaphragm (erect film?) or any obvious intra-abdominal abnormality to investigate specifically, such as distended bowel
- note tracheal position and heart size. Trace round the mediastinum and check the location of any tubes or lines. The width of the mediastinum should be noted but may be unreliable. Combined with a history suggestive of aortic aneurysm, dissection or trauma, a second opinion should be sought immediately.

## AIR BRONCHOGRAM
A bronchus is not normally visible if surrounded by aerated lung since both are equally radio-opaque. Anything that causes the normal lung tissue to lose its aerated property will produce a difference in opacity and the bronchus, provided it still contains air, will be visible. Thus, the presence of an air bronchogram suggests oedema, infection or other infiltrates in the surrounding lung tissue.

## KERLEY B LINES
These are horizontal lines that meet the pleural surface at right angles. They tend to be about 1–2 cm long and 1–2 mm thick. They are caused by increased fluid or tissue within the intralobular septa.

## BRONCHITIS AND EMPHYSEMA
Bronchitis and emphysema can be present with little or no CXR abnormalities. What may be present is increased lucency of the lung and regional or general loss of vascularity in the peripheral lung fields. The lung fields are increased in size.

## PLEURAL EFFUSION
A small effusion may only produce a blunting of the costophrenic angle. A large effusion will produce evidence of lung compression, usually respiratory problems, and the mediastinum may be displaced to the opposite side and the diaphragm flattened on that side. It is important to be aware that, with an X-ray taken with the patient supine, an effusion may show only as a faint diffuse opacity spread over the lung field. This is because the fluid is spread thinly over a wide area. Repeat the X-ray with the patient having been sat up for 15 minutes or obtain an ultrasound scan. An effusion due to a cardiac disorder tends to be bilateral.

## CONSOLIDATION
Consolidation will not produce a mediastinal shift unless there is significant collapse when the mediastinum will be drawn over to the side of the lesion.

## PERICARDIAL EFFUSION
There are many reasons for an enlarged cardiac silhouette, which can be apparent or pathological.

The most common pathological reasons include ventricular hypertrophy, pericardial effusion and ventricular aneurysm. An effusion may produce an outline that is globular in appearance but hypertrophy of the left ventricle can do the same. Left atrial enlargement can produce a straightening of the left cardiac border. A significant pericardial effusion is likely to produce evidence of tamponade with poor cardiac function and raised central venous pressure. If in doubt, ultrasound will confirm the diagnosis.

Cardiac failure may give rise to a variety of signs including upper lobe blood diversion, cardiomegaly, pleural effusions, Kerley B lines and parenchymal shadowing (diffuse or hilar 'bat's-wing').

## MANAGEMENT OF RESPIRATORY FAILURE AND COMPROMISE

The treatment plan for managing respiratory failure follows a step-wise increase/decrease in support depending on its severity (Fig. 4.4).

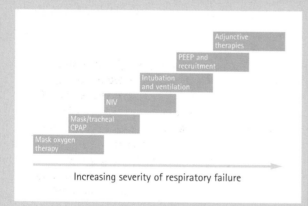

Increasing severity of respiratory failure

Figure 4.4 Treatment plan for managing respiratory failure.

During initiation of treatment, you start at the left of the scale and progress to the right as determined by your assessment of the patient's response.

Only conventional mask oxygen therapy is possible on the majority of surgical wards. Fixed delivery oxygen masks are available up to an inspired oxygen concentration of 60%, an $FiO_2$ of 0.6. All oxygen delivery systems should be humidified. Otherwise the dry, cold gas, may contribute towards thickening of the patient's secretions and promote sputum retention. Nebulised 0.9% saline (with bronchodilators if indicated) and regular

treatment from a respiratory physiotherapist may prevent worsening of incipient respiratory failure if they are used early.

The response of the patient is assessed according to the improvement of clinical status, oxygen saturation and ABG analyses. If the patient's condition does not improve with increased inspired oxygen concentration up to 60%, then you have a very unstable patient and further diagnosis and definitive treatment are required. This will involve expert help and the safe transfer of the patient to a higher level of care.

Even if the patient responds to supplemental oxygen therapy and the ABG's improve, you must remember that oxygen is only one aspect of treatment – you must treat the underlying cause of the respiratory failure.

### TREAT THE CAUSE OF RESPIRATORY FAILURE

Supportive and definitive treatments are needed. Use appropriate antibiotics, physiotherapy, diuretics, bronchodilators and cardiac or other drugs as necessary. Basal signs may indicate continuing abdominal pathology (e.g. subphrenic abscess). Systemic factors influence respiratory function (e.g. mobility, nutrition) – it is important to treat these too.

Review the patient's requirement for and response to analgesia; either too little or too much can be a factor in preventing adequate clearance of secretions by inhibiting coughing and by limiting the patient's tolerance of physiotherapy. Where sputum clearance is the primary problem, a mini-tracheostomy should be considered. Do not assume that confusion or depressed level of consciousness are due to the effects of opiate analgesia. Hypoxia may cause an acute confusional state and hypercarbia may lead to obtundation.

## RE-ASSESS

Detect failure of improvement or deterioration: persisting or worsening signs and symptoms of respiratory failure necessitate further immediate management and safe transfer to a higher level of care.

## DETECTING SIMPLE OXYGEN FAILURE

It is essential to be alert to this situation as it is common, can be rapidly fatal and requires a prompt change in management.

### FAILURE OF MASK OXYGEN THERAPY AT HIGH $FiO_2$ MAY BE INDICATED BY:

- increasing respiratory rate
- increasing distress, dyspnoea, exhaustion, sweating and confusion
- oxygen saturation 80% or less (this may be a late sign)
- $PaO_2$ less than 8 kPa
- $PaCO_2$ greater than 7 kPa.

### CASE SCENARIO 4.2

A 62-year-old woman with chronic bronchitis is 4 days postoperative following a right abdominal nephrectomy. This morning she was noted to be tachypnoeic, pyrexial and with reduced air entry, bronchial breathing and dullness to percussion at the right lung base. Her $FiO_2$ was increased to 0.8 in order to maintain $SaO_2$ above 97%. The physiotherapist obtained a sample of foul sputum for culture and antibiotics were prescribed for pneumonia. A CXR showed typical localised changes at the right base. It is now 7 p.m. and the HDU nurse has called you because she is again tachypnoeic and hypoxic despite the therapy above. Chest signs are unchanged but she is noticeably sweaty and starting to look tired. She is not in pain and, on detailed review, there does not seem to be anything else you can do to improve matters. Recent blood gases show that the $PaCO_2$ has risen from 4 kPa to 7.3 kPa over the last 10 h. The HDU nurse is experienced and worried that the patient might suddenly tire and arrest. You accept her advice and ask for an urgent ICU review. The ICU consultant is pleased that you called at this stage. CPAP on HDU is considered but the patient is hypercarbic and it is decided to take her to ICU for intubation and ventilation.

#### LEARNING POINTS

- use your routine ward rounds to monitor progress systematically but re-assess and hand over patients who are not right at the end of the routine day
- detect patients who are failing to respond or deteriorating despite reasonable therapy and refer promptly
- clinical signs (e.g. tiredness and sweating) are also important in detecting the patient at risk of respiratory failure and arrest.

The clinical signs and blood gas analysis are the most important factors. Tachypnoeic patients suddenly tire and arrest. You must intervene before this stage by acting on early symptoms and signs, particularly tachypnoea. Transfer the patient to a higher level of care for further therapy to improve gas exchange. An arterial line should be inserted if frequent blood gas analysis is to be performed. Anticipate problems in patients with severe chronic lung disease (e.g. vital capacity less than 15 ml/kg or $FEV_1$ less than 10 ml/kg) and monitor them closely.

## CONTINUOUS POSITIVE AIRWAY PRESSURE

If the primary problem is Type I respiratory failure, CPAP by mask may help. A high flow source of oxygen-enriched air is supplied through a tight-fitting facemask with a range of expiratory valves (Fig. 4.5). These valves maintain a set airway pressure, which can range from 2.5–10 $cmH_2O$. During ventilation, airway pressure cannot drop below the pressure indicated on the valve. This leads to recruitment of underventilated alveolae, increases FRC, decreases intrapulmonary shunt and may improve oxygenation.

The masks are uncomfortable to wear, may cause nasal pressure sores and, if air-swallowing occurs, result in gastric dilatation and regurgitation. Some patients unable to tolerate a full-face mask may tolerate a nasal mask but the patient must keep their mouth closed to prevent loss of pressure. CPAP may also be connected directly via a T-piece to a pre-existing tracheostomy tube. The patient must have a reasonable respiratory rate and tidal volume, be in control of his or her own airway and able to co-operate. Patients who fail to tolerate CPAP are recognised by refractory hypoxaemia, increasing respiratory rate and progressively smaller tidal volumes with subsequent $CO_2$ retention.

Patient selection is key to the success of CPAP. Frequent monitoring of the clinical status of the patient is required, including regular ABGs, within an HDU environment. A plan should be made of how frequently CPAP is to be used and for what length of time. Generally, to be beneficial, a minimum of 2 hours of continuous CPAP is required. CPAP may also be used as part of the weaning process from formal ventilation or, alternatively, used post-extubation if the patient has a high risk of re-intubation.

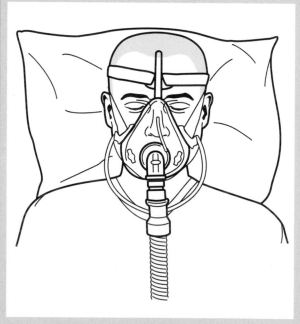

Figure 4.5 Diagramtic representation of patient receiving CPAP therapy.

## NON-INVASIVE VENTILATION BY MASK (BIPAP)

If Type II respiratory failure ($CO_2$ retention) develops, NIV support by mask should be considered. Essentially, two different pressures are applied to the patient via a facemask – a higher one during inspiration (around 20 $cmH_2O$) and a lower one in expiration (5 $cmH_2O$). This may be termed BiLevel or BIPAP mask ventilation. The pressure difference generates gas flow into the lungs during inspiration.

The BIPAP machine detects inspiration by the initial drop in airway pressure that occurs. It then automatically raises the pressure to that set on the machine for inspiration and changes back to the lower level on expiration. The tidal volume delivered is determined by the lung compliance, duration of inspiration and the driving pressure. This method of respiratory support may pre-empt the requirement for intubation and ventilation and requires critical care support. It is not effective in all patients and, as with CPAP, careful selection is required. It is not appropriate for patients who are cardiovascularly unstable, who have decreased level of consciousness, have a severe metabolic acidosis or have poor respiratory rates. Patients must be in control of their own airway and able to co-operate. Patients who fail to tolerate mask ventilation are recognised by refractory hypoxaemia, increasing respiratory rate and progressively smaller tidal volumes with worsening $CO_2$ retention. In general terms, if the patient's $CO_2$ has not improved within 30 minutes, mask ventilation is unlikely to succeed.

## VENTILATION

Intubation and ventilation allows oxygen concentrations of up to 100% and the volume of each breath (tidal volume, Vt) and respiratory rate or frequency (f) to be adjusted to suit the patient's needs. The minute volume (MV = Vt x f) may be varied by altering the frequency or tidal volume. The greater the MV, the greater the removal of carbon dioxide, but too large a tidal volume may cause barotrauma. 'Controlled mandatory ventilation' requires a fully sedated patient to tolerate the presence of the tracheal tube and the compulsory positive pressure breaths from the ventilator. This mode of ventilation allows the patient to play no part in breathing and is rarely used. Most commonly, a synchronised intermittent mandatory ventilation (SIMV) mode is used to try and preserve some of the patient's respiratory muscle activity by synchronising ventilation around the patient's own respiratory efforts.

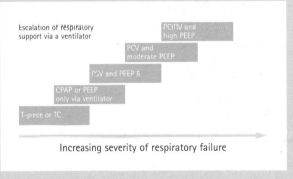

Figure 4.6 There are numerous modes of ventilatory support. The balance needs to be reached between adequate gas exchange and prevention of complications associated with artificial ventilation.

Ventilators are increasingly sophisticated and offer different forms of ventilation, which may be used in combination (Fig. 4.6). With modern modes of ventilation, such as combining SIMV with pressure control (PCV), pressure support (PSV) and positive end expiratory pressure (PEEP), there is much less need for sedation and paralysis. Generally, only the most difficult patients to ventilate should require paralysis and then only for short periods until control is achieved.

With PEEP, pressure is administered during expiration to prevent airway collapse and recruit underventilated alveoli. Lung compliance, Vt and how fast the Vt is 'pushed' into the patient determine the pressure reached within the airways at the end of each breath from the ventilator. This peak airway pressure can have adverse consequences. The intrathoracic pressure is always positive on inspiration during ventilation. This causes decreased venous return and a fall in cardiac output, which may be very severe if the patient is hypovolaemic. PEEP can exacerbate this problem. Furthermore, high values of peak airway pressure and PEEP predispose to barotrauma, which can result in tension pneumothorax.

High pressures plus high oxygen concentrations may also promote the toxic effects of oxygen; consequently, concentrations of oxygen greater than 80% are rarely used and then only for the shortest time possible. Peak airway pressures of greater than 35 $cmH_2O$ and the use of large tidal volumes cause overdistension of alveoli and damage to vascular endothelial tight junctions. This process of volutrauma promotes alveoli and vascular damage resulting in fluid leak and worsening of lung compliance. This, in turn, predisposes to even higher airway pressures.

Pressure control allows a breath to be administered to a set pressure, kept below 35 $cmH_2O$; the tidal volume then depends on the patient's lung compliance. By preventing high peak pressures, the risk of barotrauma is reduced. With pressure support, the ventilator senses that the patient has taken an inspiration and administers pressure to provide a higher tidal volume. The aim is not to achieve a normal ABG but to provide adequate

ventilation without causing barotrauma. Usual Vt is 10–12 ml/kg but much lower volumes (6–8 ml/kg) are used when ventilating. This leads to a higher $PaCO_2$, termed permissive hypercapnia. The $CO_2$ is allowed to rise as long as the pH is above 7.2. This reduces 'ventilator-induced lung injury' and is associated with improved survival (termed 'lung protective ventilatory strategy'), though clearly, if lung compliance is very poor, the $CO_2$ may rise too high.

Lung recruitment strategies such as PEEP must be combined with regular physiotherapy, suction and turning the patient to prevent alveolar collapse. CXR, ultrasonography or fibre-optic bronchoscopy should be used to identify any lung collapse amenable to bronchoscopic re-inflation, pleural effusions or undiagnosed pneumothoraces.

Normally, the ventilator is set to provide less time for inspiration than expiration. If the lungs are very poorly compliant and 'stiff', the inspiratory time may be increased to be equal or even longer than the expiratory time. This process is known as adjusting the inspiratory to expiratory (I:E) ratio. The I:E ratio may thus be normal (1:2 or 1:3), equal (1:1) or inverse (2:1). Applying a limited pressure for a prolonged period of time aims to improve gas exchange by opening the poorly compliant alveoli, holding them open for as long as possible to maximise gas exchange at pressures that will not cause barotrauma, volutrauma or decrease cardiac output.

A patient on pressure controlled inverse ratio ventilation (PCIRV), a high $FiO_2$ of > 0.8, PEEP > 10 $cmH_2O$ and permissive hypercarbia who fails to achieve oxygen saturation of greater than 85% is very likely to die. Death will occur from multiple organ failure as tissue oxygen delivery fails to meet demand. At this point, the use of an $FiO_2$

of 1.0 is justified and other adjuncts to ventilation considered. The most commonly used is to turn the patient from the supine to prone position. Redistribution of blood flow to the less consolidated or collapsed, more easily ventilated, anterior portions of the lung may result in improved oxygenation. Finally, ECLS with veno–venous cardiopulmonary bypass could be considered. None of these adjuncts to oxygenation have been shown to improve survival in prospective, randomised, controlled trials in adults: survival depends on adequate treatment of the underlying cause of organ failure.

## WEANING FROM VENTILATORY SUPPORT

Whatever the method of mechanical ventilatory support used, if treatment of the underlying cause of respiratory failure has been successful, then the patient must be 'weaned' from the ventilator (*i.e.* returned to spontaneous respiration in a safe, controlled manner). As soon as patients are able to participate in ventilation, they should be encouraged to do so as prolonged ventilation will lead to atrophy of the respiratory muscles. The various modes of ventilation can be used to allow a gradual reduction in the amount of work performed by the ventilator and an increase in the respiratory effort of the patient.

In general, it is unwise to attempt weaning until:
- the original cause of respiratory failure has been treated successfully
- sedative drugs have been reduced to a level where they will not depress respiration
- a low inspired oxygen concentration (40%) maintains a normal $PaO_2$
- $CO_2$ elimination is no longer a problem
- sputum production is minimal
- nutritional status, minerals, trace elements are normal

- neuromuscular function of the diaphragm and intercostals is adequate
- the patient is reasonably co-operative.

Most commonly used 'step-down' modes are SIMV, ASB or pressure support ventilation, often again used in combination. Alternatively, a simple T-piece may be used for periods of time allowing the patient to do all the breathing before being put back on mechanical ventilation when they show objective signs of diminished respiratory effort. The ventilator can be set to simply compensate for the presence of the tube (tube compensation, TC). The periods of time spent breathing spontaneously are increased until extubation is possible. In the majority of critical care units, a combined approach is used with PCV → SIMV → ASB/PSV → CPAP and T-piece followed by extubation. Patients may fail extubation as a result of poor airway control, laryngeal oedema, poor cough, sputum retention or simple fatigue.

## DISCHARGE FROM ICU

The period following ICU discharge is critical. In particular, when transfer occurs to a general ward without a period in HDU, the patient has to adapt to reduced levels of nursing care, physiotherapy and monitoring. A discharge summary and suggested treatment plan will usually accompany patients as they leave ICU but it is important that this is understood by the ward staff and is implemented directly. Experience shows that this does not happen automatically! This period of care exemplifies the importance of good personal communication and organisation – communication between ICU and surgical staff, between surgical and ward staff, of clear written instructions and repeated assessment of the patient. Apart from clinical re-assessment, ensure that medications have been changed to ward format and started, arrange out-of-hours physiotherapy as needed, check the oxygen concentration needed and ensure that any monitoring such as pulse oximetry is available on the ward. Speak to the on-call team and ask for formal review of the patient during the evening. If the patient does deteriorate, contact the ICU staff at an early stage; usually, attention to the details of care and ensuring they actually happen will prevent this.

## COMMON SURGICAL RESPIRATORY PROBLEMS

### ATELECTASIS
Atelectasis is defined as an absence of gas from all or part of the lung. It is commonly seen in surgical patients, particularly following abdominal and thoracic procedures. Reduced lung expansion from pain and splinting leads to retention of secretions and distal airway collapse. This is exacerbated in the elderly, overweight, smokers and those with pre-existing lung disease.
It should be anticipated in these patient groups and prevented by pre-operative breathing exercises to improve expansion, intra-operative care with humidification, ensuring good tidal volumes and avoiding unnecessarily high $FiO_2$. It can develop rapidly, if unrecognised, into respiratory failure.

The symptoms of atelectasis are cough, chest pain or breathing difficulty, low oxygen saturations, pleural effusion (transudate) and cyanosis (late sign) or tachycardia. Diagnosis is made by CXR. Generally, the white cell count (WCC) and C-reactive protein (CRP) levels remain in the normal range, though it may rise with super-imposed pneumonia. The mainstay of treatment is physiotherapy, focusing on deep breathing, encouraging coughing, and effective analgesia. An incentive spirometer is often used as part of the breathing exercises. Mobilisation should also be encouraged to improve lung inflation. Some may benefit from the use of CPAP. Antibiotics are given for additional infection.

### PNEUMONIA
Pneumonia is parenchymal or alveolar inflammation and abnormal alveolar filling with fluid (consolidation and exudation). In surgical patients, pneumonia is usually bacterial or chemical secondary to aspiration. Symptoms include cough, chest pain, fever and difficulty in breathing.

Physical examination of the lungs may be normal but often shows decreased expansion of the chest on the affected side, bronchial breathing or crackles. Percussion may be dulled over the affected lung. CXR, WCC, CRP and sputum and blood cultures all help in diagnosis.

Hospital-acquired pneumonia is more likely to be due to resistant bacteria such as MRSA, *Pseudomonas* spp., *Enterobacter* spp. and *Serratia* spp. Ventilator-associated pneumonia (VAP) is a subset of hospital-acquired pneumonia and occurs after 48 hours of mechanical ventilation. Aspiration pneumonia is caused by aspirating oral or gastric contents and may occur on induction of anaesthesia. Material aspirated may contain anaerobic bacteria leading to a secondary infective pneumonia. Treatment depends upon the clinical classification of pneumonia and also the known bacterial resistances within each hospital. Local microbiological advice should be sought.

Patients with pneumonia have a high risk of developing respiratory failure and may trigger ARDS, which results from a combination of infection and inflammatory response. The lungs quickly fill with fluid and become very stiff. This stiffness, combined with severe difficulties extracting oxygen due to the alveolar fluid, creates a requirement for mechanical ventilation.

The **CURB 65** score is frequently used when looking at severity of pneumonia: Confusion; Urea > 7 mmol/l; Respiratory rate $\geq$ 30 per min; Blood pressure (SBP < 90 mmHg or DBP $\leq$ 60 mmHg); age $\geq$ 65 years. If three or more of these factors are present, critical care admission is very likely to be required.

## PULMONARY EMBOLISM

Pulmonary embolism comprises embolic obstruction of a vascular branch beyond the right ventricular outflow tract, usually from an associated deep vein thrombosis. They are still relatively common in surgical practice, though thromboprophylactic measures reduce the risk substantially.

Common symptoms include dyspnoea, pleuritic chest pain, cough, haemoptysis and palpitations, while signs include hypoxia, tachypnoea and tachycardia. Diagnosis is based on these clinical findings in combination with laboratory tests and imaging studies. The gold standard for diagnosis is pulmonary angiography but CT pulmonary angiography is more commonly used (Fig. 4.7). CXR may be helpful in excluding other causes of deterioration. ABGs may show hypoxia and hypocarbia. The most common ECG change, apart from sinus tachycardia, is T-wave inversion in the anterior leads and echocardiography may be very useful in the unstable patient to look for right heart dysfunction.

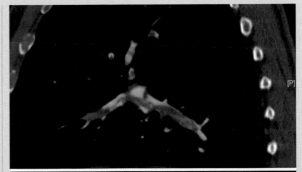

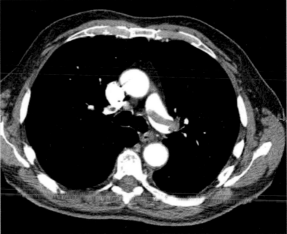

Figure 4.7 CTPA showing a saddle embolus and substantial thrombus burden in the lobar branches of both main pulmonary arteries.

## TREATMENT

In most cases, anticoagulant therapy is the mainstay of treatment. Usually, low molecular weight heparin is administered initially, prior to warfarin therapy. In the peri-operative patient, treatment is complicated by the risk of bleeding. If the risk of bleeding is high, unfractionated heparin by infusion may be used with close monitoring of APTT and monitoring of cardiovascular status and haemoglobin may be more appropriate. Alternatives include inferior vena caval filter and pulmonary embolectomy.

If there is a concern regarding bleeding, heparin can be stopped with its effect reversing within 3 hours; alternatively, it can be reversed with protamine if a more immediate effect is required.

## PRACTICAL SKILL: CHEST DRAINS

Chest drains are either inserted for pneumothorax or for drainage of pleural fluid. There are two main types of drain in common use. Seldinger-type chest drains are most frequently used for drainage of pleural effusions and small pneumothoraces, while more traditional drains are inserted for larger pneumothoraces (Fig. 4.8). The size of the chest drain used depends on the indication: a large bore tube (28–30F) should be used for haemothorax, large and/or tension pneumothorax and a smaller calibre tube (10–14F) for pleural effusions. Maintenance of patency of chest drains is important for safety; frequently, larger tubes are inserted if there is any doubt. However, larger chest drains are associated with increased pain.

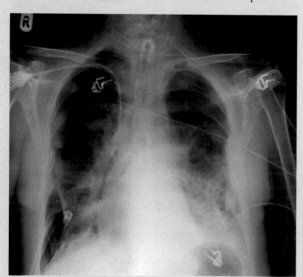

Figure 4.8 Chest X-ray showing chest drain in area of partially resolved R-sided pneumothorax.

The technique of chest drain insertion is not taught on the CCrISP course. However, surgical trainees should be able to recognise the indications, methods and complications associated with chest drainage.

All chest drains should be monitored for swinging, draining and bubbling. Chest drains should be removed as soon as they are no longer required, *i.e.* a pleural effusion drained to dryness (remember about 100–150 ml of pleural fluid is normally produced per day) or the pneumothorax is fully inflated. Caution must be used when patients are ventilated (including CPAP and NIV) as re-accumulation of pneumothorax is common and these may well be tension pneumothoraces. If a patient has a pneumothorax, generally any central line required should be put in that side to prevent the occurrence of bilateral pneumothorax. Chest drains should never be clamped.

### SUMMARY
- assess respiratory function in all ward patients who have undergone major surgery and use simple measures liberally to prevent major respiratory compromise
- routine assessment is predominantly clinical and aims to identify the patient who is deteriorating
- use the system of assessment to identify clinically those patients with respiratory failure
- instigate the level of treatment appropriate to the severity of failure
- treat the cause of the failure as well as hypoxia/hypercarbia
- re-assess clinical signs, oximetry and, most importantly, ABGs
- arrange safe transfer to higher level of care for those who do not respond.

# 5

Arterial blood
gases and
acid–base balance

## INTRODUCTION

ABG measurements are important in the management of critically ill surgical patients as they can provide a guide to acid–base status, ventilation and global tissue perfusion, plus potential compensatory mechanisms. Acid–base status is expressed via pH, ventilation through the partial pressures of oxygen and carbon dioxide and tissue perfusion via base-excess/base-deficit. Examining the trends of thesevalues in the critically ill allows clinicians to analyse the severity of a deterioration or effectiveness of their management plans. Abnormalities in ABGs may arise before a patient becomes obviously unwell and thus provide clinicians with the opportunity for early, effective intervention.

ABG samples are obtained by either arterial puncture (usually the radial artery) or from an arterial line (a-line; see Chapter 8). The complication rates of such a procedure are low but include bleeding and haematoma formation (particularly in coagulopathic patients), distal ischaemia and pseudo-aneurysm formation (the latter usually as a consequence of infected in-dwelling catheters). The techniques, risks and complications of intravascular line placement are discussed in Chapter 8. With respect to radial artery puncture, the use of Allen's test to demonstrate flow through the ulnar artery theoretically ensures that ischaemic damage will not occur due to collateral circulation; in practice, for radial blood gas sampling it is rarely used and the incidence of digital ischaemia is low.

The arterial partial pressure of oxygen ($PaO_2$) is a reflection of the amount of oxygen dissolved in the blood. Its relationship with the oxygen saturation of haemoglobin ($SaO_2$) is affected by factors such as temperature, partial pressure of carbon dioxide ($PaCO_2$) and pH, which is reflected by the oxygen dissociation curve (Fig. 5.1). The $PaO_2$ can be used as an indicator of the pressure gradient that has the potential to drive oxygen into the tissues. A normal (or supra-normal) value does not necessarily ensure effective oxygen utilisation by tissue but it does reflect adequate management of oxygen delivery by the respiratory and cardiovascular systems.

Regardless of what other ABG values show, hypoxia should be treated with oxygen therapy. A small group of patients with severe COPD rely on hypoxaemia to drive their ventilation, and high inspired oxygen concentrations ($FiO_2$) may suppress ventilation and cause hypercapnia. However, clinical progress and serial ABG measurement can assist in the management of these patients; trainees should always seek appropriate advice and help if unsure about the potential for causing hypercapnia.

## PRACTICE POINT

*While hypercapnia can kill slowly, hypoxaemia will kill quickly! Additionally, when interpreting the $PaO_2$, the $FiO_2$ should be noted and clinicians should always be aware of relative hypoxaemia, i.e. an absolute $PaO_2$ may be within 'normal limits' (10–14 kPa) but the amount of supplementary oxygen and ventilatory support may be high. A more effective means of assessing for relative hypoxaemia is the $PaO_2$:$FiO_2$ ratio, whereby a ratio of < 40 kPa is deemed hypoxic. Remember that, as the $FiO_2$ increases towards 1.0, the $PaO_2$ should increase – an oxygen saturation of 100% and $PaO_2$ of 13 kPa indicates good oxygenation for an individual breathing air ($FiO_2$ 0.21, $PaO_2$:$FiO_2$ ratio 61.9 kPa) but not necessarily for a patient on high flow oxygen (ratio 13 if the $FiO_2$ is 100%). Note also that pulse oximetry does not measure $CO_2$ and, therefore, reflects effective oxygenation rather than effective ventilation; ABGs provide a better overall picture of the ventilatory process (see below).*

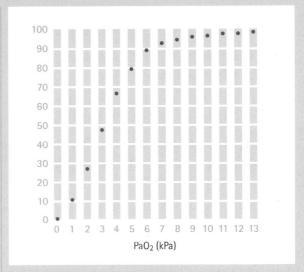

Figure 5.1 The oxygen dissociation curve.

Metabolic activity in body tissue produces energy (heat), carbon dioxide and acid, which reduces the affinity of oxygen for haemoglobin; thus, for a given $PaO_2$, oxygen is less tightly bound to haemoglobin enhancing its off-loading into cells. As this occurs, 2,3-diphosphoglycerate (2,3-DPG) present in red blood cells further loosens the bonds between haemoglobin and oxygen. The reverse is the case in the lungs, resulting in increased binding between haemoglobin and oxygen.

## INTERPRETING AN ARTERIAL BLOOD GAS

A simple sequential approach to interpreting ABGs can allow a doctor to detect abnormalities, basic pathophysiological processes (metabolic versus respiratory) and compensatory mechanisms of any acid–base disturbance. Approximate normal ranges for ABG components are outlined overleaf.

## NORMAL RANGES FOR ABG COMPONENTS

**pH:** normal range 7.35–7.45. Outlines whether a pathophysiological process has created an acidaemia or alkalaemia.

**$PaCO_2$:** normal range 4.5–5.5 kPa. This provides information about the absolute ventilatory state of a patient and possible respiratory compensatory mechanisms.

**$HCO_3^-$:** normal range 24–28 mmol/l. Bicarbonate is the main plasma buffer; a low value suggests consumption often due to increase acid-load (invariably lactic acid) and a high value suggests retention of base to compensate for hypoventilation causing an acidaemia (see below).

**Base deficit/base excess:** normal range +2 to –2 mmol/l. This describes whether the body's buffers are being consumed (deficit) or retained (excess).

**$PaO_2$:** normal range 10–14 kPa. Outlines the level of oxygenation (taking into account the $FiO_2$).

**Serum lactate:** normal range < 1.2 mmol/l. This is primarily a reflection of the extent of anaerobic metabolism occurring within the body and secondarily a reflection of the liver's ability to metabolise lactate and regenerate bicarbonate anions.

**The anion gap:** normal range 10–15 mmol/l. Plasma exists in electrochemical neutrality, *i.e.* the number of cations and anions balance; however, the majority of laboratory assays measure approximately 95% of cations and 85% of anions creating a differential described as the anion gap or AG.

$$AG = ([Na^+] + [K^+]) - ([Cl^-] + [HCO_3^-])$$

The majority of 'unmeasured anions' are plasma proteins but also include small concentrations of phosphate, sulphate and organic acids. An acidaemia with an increase in the anion gap indicates an increase in the concentration of these unmeasured anions (*e.g.* lactate and ketones). An acidaemia with a normal anion gap equates to the total concentration of measured anions being unchanged usually as a consequence of hyperchloraemic acidaemia. This is most frequently seen following vigorous resuscitation with 0.9% saline but is also associated with bladder surgery and ileal conduit formation.

## ACID–BASE BALANCE

The concentration of hydrogen ions within the body is normally tightly controlled at 40 nmol/l, which is 7.42 pH units (pH = $-\log_{10}[H^+]$).

Over 1000 mmol of hydrogen ion is produced per day, primarily as a result of the production of carbon dioxide. This is excreted by the lung and is dependent upon the minute ventilation as controlled by chemoreceptors in the medulla. There is also a smaller quantity of hydrogen ion produced as non-volatile acid products of metabolism of non-carbohydrate substrate, such as phosphates and sulphates. This amounts to approximately 1 mmol $H^+$/kg/day and must be excreted by the distal nephron. There are, therefore, two control mechanisms maintaining hydrogen ion homeostasis – respiratory and renal.

The respiratory mechanism is a rapid-response system that requires normal CNS function (central pH chemoreceptors) and lung function to allow carbon dioxide to be transferred from pulmonary venous blood to alveolar gas and excreted in expired gas. Any dysfunction of the mechanics or control of respiration will cause retention of $CO_2$ and a rise in hydrogen ion concentration (respiratory acidosis) or over-excretion and a fall in hydrogen ion concentration (respiratory alkalosis).

The renal mechanism is a slower responding system that depends upon the excretion of hydrogen ions in the urine by the distal nephron. Conditions that impair renal function and, in particular, distal nephron function (e.g. obstructive uropathy, circulating volume depletion) will prevent non-volatile hydrogen ion excretion resulting in a metabolic acidosis.

The body's homeostatic mechanisms with regard to the maintenance of acid–base balance are powerful and a patient can have a normal pH in the face of marked physiological disturbance. Furthermore, as the pH scale is a log-based scale, small changes in pH represent major physiological disturbances. Proteins are the primary buffer of retained hydrogen ion; however, because of the importance of the carbon dioxide/bicarbonate system in the elimination of hydrogen ion, the acid–base status of the body is best reflected by the measurement of carbon dioxide tension and bicarbonate level in the blood. This measures both the volatile and non-volatile arms of the system.

$$(H^+) + HCO_3^- \longleftrightarrow H_2CO_3 \longleftrightarrow H_2O + CO_2$$

Non-volatile           Volatile

(Renal)             (Respiratory)

### RESPIRATORY ACIDOSIS

The retention of carbon dioxide will cause a rise of $H^+$ by driving the acid-base equation to the left. The kidney will respond slowly over approximately 48 hours to compensate by increasing $H^+$ excretion in the distal nephron, thus returning $H^+$ concentration toward, but not completely, normal.

### METABOLIC ACIDOSIS

The inability of the kidney to excrete non-volatile hydrogen ion or a sudden increase in non-volatile acid load (such as in sepsis) will drive the equation to the right and respiratory function will rapidly respond by increasing minute volume, reduce CO2 and cause hydrogen ion to return toward normal.

## RESPIRATORY ALKALOSIS

Respiratory alkalosis is caused by the minute ventilation being higher than that required to maintain the $PaCO_2$ appropriate for a hydrogen ion concentration of 40 nmol/l. The $PaCO_2$ is driven down and the hydrogen ion falls (pH rises). This is usually caused by an increased central respiratory drive commonly by fever, hepatic disease, aspirin toxicity or CNS dysfunction.

## METABOLIC ALKALOSIS

Metabolic alkalosis occurs when the level of bicarbonate in the blood is increased due either to abnormal retention or administration of bicarbonate or the loss of non-volatile acid from the body (gastric outlet obstruction or chronic nasogastric aspiration). Abnormal retention of bicarbonate can occur in association with chloride depletion due to loop diuretics and is also seen in chronic hypokalaemia.

Knowing the hydrogen ion concentration/pH, $PaCO_2$ and bicarbonate allows the acid–base status to be determined, thus the type of abnormality and degree of compensation to be estimated. The most useful bicarbonate measure is the standardised value, which corrects the measured bicarbonate to the value that would be present if the $PaCO_2$ was normal (40 mmHg or 5.4 kPa). The non-volatile acid–base state is also summarised by the calculated base excess, which gives a value of the difference between the standardised bicarbonate and the normal value. This is otherwise considered as the amount of acid or alkali needed to return blood *in vivo* to normal pH under standard conditions.

# THE MANAGEMENT OF ACID–BASE DISTURBANCE

The first step is to manage the patient according to CCrISP principles and then investigate the nature of the disturbance using ABG samples and other investigations relevant to the patient's history. The importance of determining the underlying primary disturbance can point the clinician towards definitive treatment of an underlying problem. While this is achieved, measures may be required for temporary correction of the pH by other means. Examples of aetiologies and case histories are illustrated below:

### AETIOLOGY OF COMMON ACID–BASE DISTURBANCES

Metabolic acidosis
- impaired tissue perfusion – deal with cause, improve circulation/perfusion
- renal failure – deal with cause, bicarbonate, renal replacement therapy
- hepatic failure – ?transplant.

Respiratory acidosis
- head or spinal injury – ventilation
- drug overdose – antidote (*e.g.* Naloxone) and/or ventilation if indicated
- chest wall deformity or injury – ventilation if indicated
- myopathy or peripheral neuropathy – ventilation if indicated
- pulmonary disease – treat disease, respiratory support and ventilation if indicated
- massive pulmonary embolus – re-establish perfusion of ventilated lung.

## EXAMPLES OF ACID–BASE DISTURBANCE IN CLINICAL PRACTICE

### CASE 1

A 54-year-old man, 14 h post-laparoscopic hemicolectomy, receiving oxygen at 4 l/min via a facemask and using a morphine PCA. Respiratory rate is 8 breaths/min.
ABGs:
pH, 7.24
$PaCO_2$, 9.8 kPa
$PaO_2$, 15.1 kPa
$HCO_3^-$, 24.2 mmol/l
BE, +0.2 mmol/l
Lactate, 0.9 mmol/l

**What is the nature of the blood gas abnormality and how should you manage the situation?**

This is an uncompensated respiratory acidaemia, most probably caused by excess opiate. Oxygenation remains good; however, in time, the patient will become hypoxaemic without intervention. Assess using the CCrISP system with early administration of high flow oxygen and Naloxone.

### CASE 2

A 72-year-old woman with known diverticular disease presented to the surgical admissions unit with abdominal pain and peritonism. Respiratory rate is 28 breaths/min and breathing face mask oxygen at 4 l/min.
ABGs:
pH, 7.30
$PaCO_2$, 3.8 kPa
$PaO_2$, 9.1 kPa
$HCO_3^-$, 18.7 mmol/l
BE, −7.0 mmol/l
Lactate, 2.1 mmol/l

**What is the nature of the blood gas abnormality and how should you manage the situation?**

This patient has a partially compensated metabolic acidaemia and is hypoxic. She is likely to have intra-abdominal sepsis with increase acid load indicated by loss of buffer (low $HCO_3^-$) and raised serum lactate. The tachypnoea is a consequence of an attempted compensation for the acidaemia and also the likely consequence of pain, which in turn can cause diaphragmatic splinting, atelectasis, hypoxaemia and, if ineffectively managed, worsening hypercapnia. This patient requires aggressive resuscitation, analgesia and management of the source of sepsis ('source control').

### PRACTICE POINT

*Be aware of the tachypnoeic, acidaemic patient with a raised $CO_2$.*

## CASE 3

A 48-year-old man with Crohn's disease, an ileostomy and large stoma losses. He is tachypnoeic and breathing room air.
ABGs:
pH, 7.25
$PaCO_2$, 3.2kPa
$PaO_2$, 17.1 kPa
$HCO_3^-$, 14.2 mmol/l
BE, −9.9 mmol/l
Lactate, 1.0 mmol/l

## CASE 4

A 78-year-old man presents to surgical admissions 1 month after a Whipple's procedure with nausea and vomiting for the previous 3 days, and a distended abdomen.
ABGs:
pH, 7.54
$PaCO_2$, 6.7 kPa
$PaO_2$, 11.5 kPa
$HCO_3^-$, 31.5 mmol/l
BE, +4.8 mmol/l
Lactate, 0.7 mmol/l

**What is the nature of the blood gas abnormality and how should you manage the situation?**

He has a metabolic acidaemia with attempts at compensation but not effective enough to prevent a low pH. There is likely to have been large loss of bicarbonate from the stoma. In addition to CCrISP assessment, investigation and treatment of the cause, fluid replacement with a crystalloid such as Hartmann's solution is appropriate to replace many of the electrolytes being lost; furthermore, if the liver function is normal, the lactate anions can be utilised to generate bicarbonate, help replace losses and correct the acidaemia.

**What is the nature of the blood gas abnormality?**

He has a partially compensated metabolic alkalaemia, most probably secondary to loss of gastric acid through vomiting, quite possibly induced by gastric outlet obstruction.

**SUMMARY**
The interpretation of blood gases is an essential part of caring for surgical patients.
- pH indicates whether there is acidosis or alkalosis
- base excess indicates whether acidosis is metabolic (negative base excess) or respiratory
- low $PaO_2$ indicates the presence of hypoxia
- high $PaCO_2$ and acidosis (plus high $HCO_3^-$ and positive base excess) indicates respiratory acidosis
- initial management of any acid–base disturbance begins with the CCrISP algorithm.

# 6

## Cardiovascular disorders, diagnosis and management

The following three chapters deal with aspects of cardiovascular disorders, shock and monitoring and should be considered together. This first section will introduce a basic pattern of thinking that should enable the early detection of an impending cardiovascular problem. Preventative measures, simple treatments or referral to a specialist unit can then be initiated appropriately. This chapter will focus on clinical assessment and the diagnosis and management of cardiac disorders. Management and treatment of shock will be covered in Chapter 7, while more invasive monitoring and support will be detailed in Chapter 8.

Disorders of the CVS are very common in the sick surgical patient and can be due to associated medical co-morbidity or arise as complications following surgical procedures. Despite the presence of an intact airway and adequate ventilation, any problem causing decreased efficiency of the CVS can result in inadequate delivery of oxygen to the tissues for their metabolic needs. This will initiate a cascade of adverse events that will lead to the development of organ failure. The range of pathologies that cause CVS disturbance is broad, including inadequate or excessive circulating volume, primary 'pump' problems and increased or reduced afterload. While organ failure may be obvious, it more frequently presents with more subtle and gradual deteriorations in the presence of apparently 'normal' or slightly deranged pulse rates and blood pressure. Early recognition of an impending problem and initiation of effective treatment will increase your patient's chances of survival and help to prevent further complications. Prediction and prevention are vital.

For these reasons, the approach to the examination of the CVS must be systematic, accurately documented and repeated frequently. The effect of any intervention, such as fluid administration, must be re-assessed to ensure its efficacy and durability. It is also imperative to pay great attention to a patient's concurrent cardiac medications.

## PATIENT ASSESSMENT AND MANAGEMENT

### IMMEDIATE ASSESSMENT AND RESUSCITATION

To establish that the patient does not need immediate life-saving resuscitation, you need to make your immediate ABC assessment using the CCrISP algorithm. Keep an open mind; do not try and make the findings fit any preconceived diagnosis, and remember to initiate immediate and appropriate resuscitation during the assessment. Hypovolaemia due to haemorrhage or unreplaced fluid losses should be considered the primary cause of CVS dysfunction in the surgical patient until proved otherwise. Thereafter, sepsis, cardiac dysfunction or pulmonary embolism represent common problems.

The presence of dyspnoea increases the likelihood of a cardiac and/or respiratory problem. Breathing and the CVS are inextricably linked; a disorder of the respiratory system (*e.g.* tension pneumothorax) may produce CVS signs and similarly a CVS disorder (*e.g.* left ventricular failure) may produce respiratory signs.

All other organ systems are dependent on the viability of the circulation. This is particularly true of the renal and the central nervous systems, and the integrity of these end organs can give valuable information about the function of the CVS. If the patient is obtunded or too confused to respond coherently, then cerebral hypoperfusion or hypoxia is likely and prompt action will be needed.

Life-threatening CVS disorders are recognisable if you examine the patient appropriately:

- **look for:** pallor, poor peripheral perfusion, underfilled or overfilled veins, obvious blood loss from wounds, drains or stomas, swelling of soft tissues or other evidence of concealed haemorrhage into chest, abdomen or pelvis. Ankle or sacral oedema
- **listen to the patient:** confusion might be due to poor cerebral perfusion; if they say they feel faint on sitting up or are thirsty, consider hypovolaemia. A complaint of breathlessness on lying flat may point to fluid overload. Complaints of chest pain, breathlessness, feeling feverish or cold are all helpful in determining underlying pathology and should not be ignored. Listen to the chest and heart.

**PRACTICE POINT**

*Listen to the heart – normal heart sounds or gallop rhythm?*
*Is there a new murmur?*

- **feel for:** carotid and femoral pulses if peripheral radial pulses are not present. Assess for rate, quality (weak/thready/strong), regularity and equality. Examine for swelling, distension or painful areas that may indicate internal bleeding or ischaemia. Feel for changes in skin temperature and assess capillary refill.

**PRACTICE POINT**

*Unwell surgical patients will benefit from oxygen and fluid therapy while you are performing your assessment.*

## FULL PATIENT ASSESSMENT
### Chart review
The notes and charts contain a lot of data; again, a systematic approach minimises the chance of missing important facts. Sometimes, it can be useful to complete your note and chart review before speaking in detail to the ward nurses and doctors. This provides you with a factual base for discussing the patient in more detail. The notes will provide basic clinical information on pre-morbid status, co-morbidity and any procedures performed. On the charts, look at both the absolute values and the trends. Absolute values are notoriously unreliable and more useful information can be obtained by looking at trends over the preceding few hours. The charts should

indicate the progress of the patient and important parameters include:

- respiratory rate, oxygen $FiO_2$ and saturation
- heart rate and rhythm
- blood pressure – systolic/diastolic
- CVP (if measured)
- temperature
- urinary output
- i.v. lines – position and condition
- fluid therapy – prescribed versus given, drainage of all types
- review drug chart for drugs with CVS effects (given/omitted).

*Respiratory rate*
- most sensitive marker of the 'ill' patient and often the first parameter to change as the patient deteriorates
- accurate observation and recording is essential
- rates < 11 may be due to opiate/sedative overdose or other causes of CNS depression including low cardiac output
- high respiratory rate is an early sign of many kinds of shock, as well as respiratory disease or cardiac failure
- an increased respiratory rate may be in response to hypoxia and/or metabolic acidosis.

*Heart rate and rhythm*
- there is wide individual variation with age and disease
- interpret absolute values of pulse rate along with co-existing medical conditions or drug treatment: beware the patient on ß-blockers or who has a pacemaker as the normal cardiac response to hypovolaemia or pyrexia will be blocked
- tachycardia can be an early sign of shock
- acute dysrhythmia is an important sign of myocardial failure or ischaemia.

*Blood pressure*
- changes in both systolic and diastolic pressure are often late signs but, when present, should flag up the severity of the underlying problem
- think perfusion rather than pressure: a high or normal blood pressure with poor perfusion is of little benefit to the patient
- remember that for the elderly patient who usually runs at 180/100, a pressure of 110/70 represents significant hypotension.

Clinical signs may be unreliable in that normal values do not exclude significant abnormality. However, abnormal values should be acted upon!

*Jugular venous pressure/central venous pressure*
- jugular venous distension measured with the patient 45° in the sitting position will give a clinical indication of the CVP
- collapsed neck veins with the patient at 45° indicates low JVP
- JVP not visible with the patient flat is always abnormal
- the CVP response to a fluid bolus is a better guide to fluid status than absolute value
- the trend in CVP reading is a very valuable tool in assessing ongoing fluid status
- consider formal CVP monitoring early in ill patients when management of fluids is becoming problematic.

Abnormalities relating to the CVP are detailed in Table 6.1.

## TABLE 6.1

### ABNORMALITIES OF CVP

**A low CVP may be:**
- due to inadequate fluid therapy
- an indication of continued bleeding
- due to vasodilatation in response to sepsis
- may be associated with a low cardiac output
- explained by vasodilatation due to epidural analgesia – exclude other causes!
- a low CVP must be corrected in the face of hypotension.

**A high CVP may be:**
- temporary following a rapid fluid bolus
- a result of fluid overload
- due to right ventricular failure as a result of MI or pulmonary embolism
- due to CCF
- due to chronic respiratory disease
- caused by pericardial effusion with tamponade.

If in any doubt as to the cause or treatment required, seek expert help!

*Temperature*
- may be high (> 38°C) or low (< 36°C) in sepsis or SIRS but may be normal even in the presence of severe intra-abdominal sepsis in the immunocompromised, elderly or patient on steroids
- core/peripheral temperature (rectal/axillary) difference > 2°C suggests poor peripheral perfusion

- low-grade pyrexia occurs after MI in bacterial endocarditis (irregular, mild and accompanied by a cardiac murmur and anaemia) or with diurnal variation in a warm environment (highest in the early evening).

*Urinary output*
- probably the best surrogate marker of cardiac output and tissue perfusion that is readily available on the ward BUT it is not an immediate and acute measurement
- the hypoxic or underperfused kidney does not perform well and is an excellent marker of early cardiovascular problems
- look for a steady decline to indicate a problem rather than sudden complete anuria, which suggests a blocked catheter.

*Intravenous lines*
- careful aseptic management of i.v. lines is essential to avoid line sepsis
- Large-bore i.v. access is required to deliver an appropriate rapid fluid bolus
- tissued lines cause morbidity both from the local effect of extravasated fluids and drugs and, systemically, as a result of the failure of the fluid and drugs to reach the circulation. A patient with a tissued drip relying on i.v. fluids may become dehydrated quickly.

*Tubes and drains*
- may or may not be patent
- sudden occlusion of chest drains may lead to tension pneumothorax
- pericardial drains occluding after cardiac surgery may cause cardiac tamponade
- occluded abdominal drains may delay recognition of ongoing bleeding
- drainage volumes and nasogastric aspirate are an essential part of fluid balance calculations.

*Drug chart review*
- may reveal that regular cardiac drugs have been omitted while the patient was 'nil-by-mouth'
- alternatively, drugs may have been administered that have produced adverse cardiovascular effects as a result of overdosage, accumulation or interaction with other systems (*e.g.* steroids preventing pyrexia in sepsis or masking abdominal signs).

*Fluid balance*
- determine type and quantity of fluids given; the fluid balance for the current 24 hours and for the preceding days
- has the fluid been given as prescribed (often inadequate, slow or curtailed)?
- it is much more frequent for unwell surgical patients to be hypovolaemic rather than fluid overloaded
- however, pulmonary oedema may be iatrogenic, particularly in the elderly patient with a cardiac history. In these patients, fluid should be given in small repeated boluses to correct hypovolaemia
- remember that all patients are different and do not respond identically to apparently similar fluid regimens.

*History*
Taking a careful and detailed history from the patient and from the notes will help to identify cardiac problems. Remember that nursing colleagues and relatives can be useful additional sources of information. Specific points worth remembering include:
- speed of onset and duration of any symptoms
- pain, its nature, severity, site and radiations
- presence of dyspnoea
- functional exercise tolerance.

*Case notes*
The pre-admission cardiac status and medication should be identified from the notes when making an assessment of the CVS, both when complications are occurring and when the daily management plan is being formulated.

*Examination*
Utilise all the available clinical information and think perfusion. Concentrate on the CVS.

**LOOK**
- overview – is the patient alert? A reduced level of consciousness is often a clear sign of reduced cardiac output
- colour – presence of peripheral or central cyanosis; anaemia
- peripheries – assess for peripheral perfusion and presence of oedema. Assess limb temperature
- neck veins.

**LISTEN**
*Breath sounds*
- assess for the presence of basal crepitations, indicative of left-sided failure
- in early, left-sided failure, bronchial wheeze (cardiac asthma) may be present due to small airway narrowing as a result of interstitial pulmonary oedema.

*Heart sounds*
- assess for the presence of added sounds or murmurs (?new)
- time the murmur with the carotid pulse: remember a diastolic murmur is never 'physiological'.

## FEEL

- skin – may feel clammy with poor capillary filling in cardiogenic shock or warm with good capillary refill in sepsis
- liver – assess for presence of hepatomegaly or ascites which may be an indication of congestive heart failure. Heart failure can cause abdominal pain from acute distension of the liver capsule.

### TABLE 6.2

#### INDICATORS OF A LOW CARDIAC OUTPUT

Cool, clammy skin with poor capillary flushing
- Rapid, low volume pulse
- Peripheral cyanosis
- Low peripheral temperature/core. peripheral temperature gradient (> 2°C)
- Oliguria or anuria
- Confusion
- Metabolic acidaemia.

*Available results*

Include the available results and previous investigations in your assessment. Remember that ward care is different to HDU/ICU care and it is unlikely that the complete range of cardiovascular tests will have been performed. Be realistic, look at what is available and use the findings of your clinical examination, note and chart review to determine if any further specific tests are required. Demanding unnecessary tests is time consuming, costly and inflicts further discomfort to the patient. As a minimum to aid your assessment, look at the most recent haemoglobin, white cell count, platelet count and electrolyte/urea and compare them with those taken when the patient was well. If no contemporary results are available since deterioration, these will need to be ordered. Additional tests will be necessary if you suspect particular problems (*e.g.* cardiac enzymes for MI).

*Blood results*

*Haemoglobin*
- anaemia may well precipitate failure in the cardiac patient and caution will be required during transfusion. Diuretic cover may be needed (but not always – consider cardiac function and volume state)
- recent studies show that transfusions should be used to maintain a haemoglobin level around 8 g/dl
- If the patient is actively bleeding, more blood will be required.

*Electrolytes*
- potassium and magnesium are particularly important for cardiac function (see Chapter 11)
- if infarction/ischaemia is suspected, serial troponin levels should be measured from 6 hours after the onset of symptoms
- brain natriuretic peptide (BNP) levels may help in assessing heart failure.

*The chest X-ray*

The chest radiograph can help differentiate respiratory conditions from cardiovascular and aids in the positive identification of heart failure. Refer to the system for looking at radiographs in Chapter 4.

Remember chest X-rays take time and should not delay treatment. If the patient is unwell, they should not be sent to the radiology department without monitoring and the appropriate level of care.

*The electrocardiograph*
As with other investigations, the ECG should never be looked at in isolation but should be interpreted in light of the clinical findings. It may show nothing significant, even in the failing heart, but it is important to be able to recognise common patterns. Most bedside monitors do not show a trace adequate for accurate diagnosis so a formal 12-lead ECG is essential. Further instruction and practice in the interpretation of ECGs and the management of common

dysrhythmias in surgical patients will be given during the practical course.

## INTERPRETING THE ECG

### OBJECTIVES
- to learn a system for examining ECGs
- to be aware of the common important abnormalities in critically ill surgical patients
- to know the initial treatment of common cardiac dysrhythmias.

Always work to a routine when looking at an ECG (Table 6.3). Check patient name/date/time and compare with previous ECGs.

### TABLE 6.3

#### THE ROUTINE FOR LOOKING AT AN ECG

| | | |
|---|---|---|
| Axis | Use deflection in bipolar leads | |
| Rhythm | Use the R wave (lead II) | ?Regular |
| Rate | Use the R wave | ?Normal |
| P wave | Presence and morphology | ?Sinus rhythm |
| PR interval | Short<br>Long | Pre-excitation (*e.g.* WPW)<br>(*e.g.* heart block) |
| QRS complex | Height, width, presence Q waves | ?MI, ?BBB |
| ST segment | Depressed or elevated | ?MI, ?ischaemia, ?digitalis toxicity |
| T wave | Height, shape | ?Ischaemia, ?biochemical abnormalities |
| U wave | Presence | ?Hypokalaemia |

## ROTATION OF THE HEART AND MORPHOLOGY OF THE PRECORDIAL QRS COMPLEXES

The rotation of the heart determines the appearance of the QRS complexes in the different leads (Fig. 6.1). The size of the R wave in V1 increases progressively towards V6 because the underlying myocardium becomes progressively thicker over the left ventricle. Note depolarisation occurs from endocardium to epicardium and this reflects myocardial thickness. Occasionally, the R wave in V6 may be smaller than V5 and that in V5 may be smaller than V4 – this is because the electrodes in these leads are further away from the myocardium than in V1 to V3 in these cases.

The size of the S wave (first negative deflection after the R wave) tends to decrease towards V6. The direction of the first part of the QRS complex is upwards in V1 to V3 (an R wave) but this becomes a negative deflection as it progresses to V6 (Q wave). This is not pathological and is due to rotation of the heart about a near vertical axis (left hip to right shoulder), thus producing a variation in the relative positions of the two ventricles. This rotation causing the variations in QRS complexes is not clinically significant and is dependent on the individual.

Since the height of the R wave and depth of the S wave are influenced by the thickness of the underlying myocardium, these deflections will be abnormally large in conditions producing hypertrophy, for example, left ventricular hypertrophy secondary to hypertension or aortic valve disease. However, in the thin individual the R wave may be 'abnormally' high over V4 to V6.

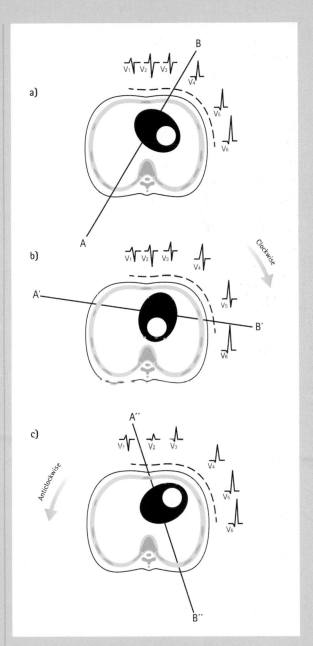

Figure 6.1 Rotation of the heart and morphology of the precordial QRS complexes. The cross section through the thorax is viewed from below. (a) intermediate position, (b) clockwise rotation, (c) anticlockwise rotation.

## THE ELECTRICAL AXIS OF THE HEART

The spread of depolarisation across the myocardium produces 'vector loops' of electrical activity. When the depolarisation wave moves towards an electrode, an upwards or positive deflection will be recorded. Conversely, moving away from an electrode will produce a downwards or negative deflection. The angle at which this electrical wave moves in relationship to a particular electrode will determine the degree of upward or downward deflection recorded by it. Each lead of the ECG 'looks' at the heart from a different aspect, or angle. These 'angles' can be displayed using the Hexaxial Reference System.

Fig. 6.2 shows the 'angle' that each bipolar lead 'sees' of the heart. By comparing the relative heights of the R wave and depth of the S wave, the electrical axis or sum of the depolarisation vectors can be determined. Basically, the more the electrical axis points towards an electrode, the greater the deflection produced by that electrode. See leads II and F in Fig. 6.2a and leads L and I in Fig. 6.2b.

This description is simplified and is only intended to give you an outline of the subject.

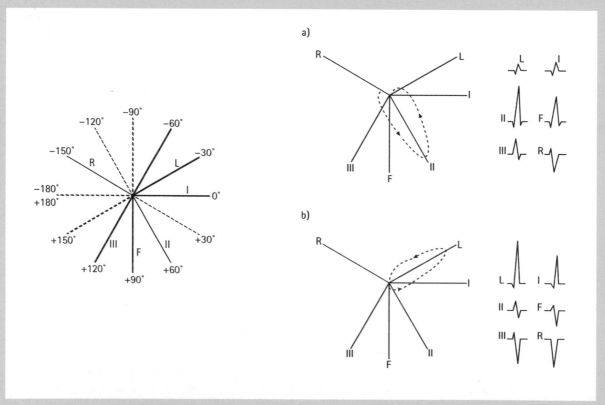

Figure 6.2 Electrical axis of the heart.

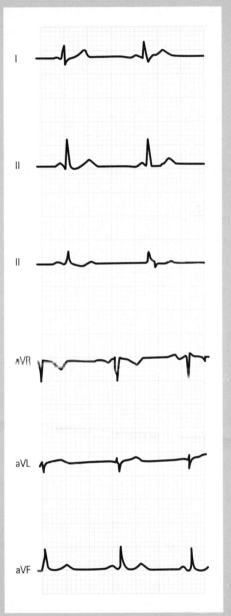

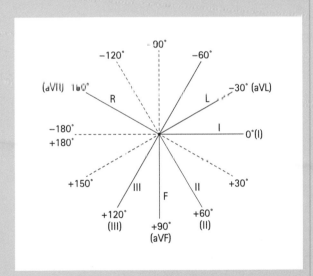

Figure 6.3 Example to demonstrate determining the electrical axis of the heart.

Look at the example provided in Fig. 6.3. Using the theory above, can you determine the electrical axis?

## TABLE 6.4

### NORMAL ECG RANGES

| | |
|---|---|
| At 25 mm/s | Large square = 0.2 s<br>Small square = 0.04 s |
| QRS width | Normal < 0.12 s<br>Wide > 0.12 s |
| Tachycardia | Is a ventricular rate > 100 bpm |
| Bradycardia | Is a ventricular rate < 60 bpm |
| Electrical axis | +90 to –30<br>Vertical +60 to +90 (tall individuals)<br>Intermediate +30 to +60<br>Horizontal +30 to –30 (stocky, squat individuals)<br>Axis shifts towards the left in the elderly |
| T wave | Normally upright, except in aVR. Inversion can also occur in III, V1 and V2 |
| P wave | Normally upright<br>Inversion can occur in retrograde P waves in AV nodal rhythm<br>Tall, peaked waves in pulmonary hypertension ('pulmonary P')<br>Biphasic in mitral valve disease ('mitral P') |
| PR interval | Measured from the start of the P wave to the first deflection of the QRS complex, whether it be upright to inverted<br>Range = 0.12–0.2 s |
| QT interval | Variable, depends on rate |
| Q wave | The first downward (negative) deflection after the P wave<br>Normal in lead III and aVR and sometimes in V4, V5, V6<br>Width no more than 0.04 s duration<br>Depth no more than one quarter the height of the following R wave |
| U wave | Normal when T wave is normal, but in hypokalaemia it may become more prominent as the T wave flattens |

## NORMAL RANGES IN ECG INTERPRETATION

The normal ranges in ECG interpretation are shown in Table 6.4 and Figs. 6.4 and 6.5.

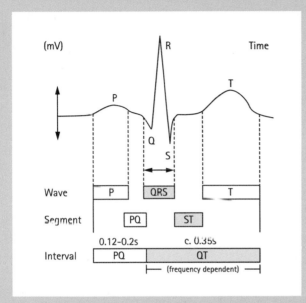

Figure 6.4 **Normal annotated PQRST.**

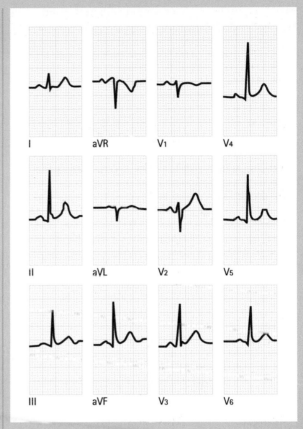

Figure 6.5 **Normal ECG trace.**

## DECIDE, PLAN AND TREAT

The clinical assessment and investigations described above should lead to a diagnosis that explains the patient's deterioration. The next task is to reach a decision based on the findings and, if needs be, arrange appropriate investigations or specialist opinions. Make a management plan to treat the problem and prevent recurrence.

Conditions that do not rapidly resolve with relatively simple measures will require expert help and a higher level of care. After any intervention you will need to re-assess and modify the management plan.

Remember the CVS has considerable reserve and, by the time dysfunction is evident, the problems are marked. Do not leave patients with obviously compromised cardiovascular systems – they won't be there when you get back!

## SPECIFIC MANAGEMENT PROBLEMS

### DIAGNOSIS AND MANAGEMENT OF HYPOTENSION

Remember that hypotension is the commonest cardiovascular problem seen in surgical critical care patients. This has been discussed in the chapter on patient assessment (Chapter 2) and will be explored further in the chapter on shock (Chapter 7).

## DIAGNOSIS AND MANAGEMENT OF TACHYARRYTHMIAS

Being called to evaluate a surgical patient with a tachycardia is common (Table 6.5). Management initially follows the system of assessment.

A patient with unstable vital signs needs prompt diagnosis and treatment. At the other end of the spectrum, long-standing, asymptomatic AF is common in the elderly and might simply need attention to fluid balance and re-institution of routine digoxin treatment. Usually, some action will be required. If any doubt exists, ask for senior help.

### TABLE 6.5

#### CAUSES OF TACHYCARDIA
(The type of tachycardia will only be evident from the ECG)

| | |
|---|---|
| Trauma | Hypovolaemia, anaemia, contused myocardium |
| Inflammatory | Pyrexia, pericarditis |
| Metabolic | Acidosis |
| Haematological | Anaemia |
| Circulatory | Shock, from any cause, arrhythmias, PE, MI |
| Endocrine | Thyrotoxicosis |
| Drugs | Aminophylline, digitalis toxicity, b-agonists |
| Anxiety and pain | |

## MANAGEMENT ALGORITHM FOR TACHYARRYTHMIAS

*Assessment*

A systematic approach to the problem should be adopted, using the CCrISP algorithm.

- check and correct ABCs – CPR or immediate anaesthetic and cardiology support may be necessary. It is better to summon help before arrest occurs
- 12-lead ECG – to allow accurate diagnosis and exclude MI
- rule out/correct: hypovolaemia, hypoxia, hypokalaemia; hypomagnesaemia
- check routine medications have been given.

*Autonomic manoeuvres*

- carotid sinus massage and Valsalva manoeuvres may correct a supraventricular tachycardia as described below but this is unlikely to be permanent.

*Drugs*

- care must be taken with all drugs, particularly in patients with poor ventricular function or hypotension
- there are various groups of drugs available for the treatment of tachyarrythmias
- if the diagnosis is not clear after clinical and ECG interpretation, the administration of adenosine can be revealing (see below)
- only use a drug if you are familiar with its actions and its side effects
- if there is any doubt about a drug, it should not be given and help must be sought early!
- remember, in the longer term, if AF or flutter persists, anticoagulation will be necessary in order to prevent emboli.

## CASE SCENARIO 6.1

A 73-year-old man, who is a known hypertensive who usually takes amlodipine, underwent anterior resection for carcinoma of the rectum this morning. You review him at 8 p.m. on the evening of surgery and find him to be in AF with a rate of 90 bpm. This developed about 30 min previously. On your immediate assessment you find that he appears quite well and tells you that he feels comfortable (he has an epidural infusion in progress). His respiratory rate is 18 breaths/min and his oxygen saturation is reading 97% with facemask oxygen at 40%. You examine him and find that his peripheries are well perfused. His blood pressure is unchanged from pre-operatively at 150/80. Your initial assessment reveals no other findings. You review his charts and notes and find that his urine output has only been 40 ml over the last 2 h. His CVP has been gradually decreasing since return from theatre and is now reading 2 mmHg. He was prescribed 2 units of blood to run over 3 h each, followed by 1000 ml saline 8-hourly by the anaesthetist. The first litre of saline has just been started. You ask the nurse to give him the litre of saline over 1 h, and check a full blood count and his urea and electrolytes. His haemoglobin is satisfactory at 11.0 g/dl. His serum potassium is 3.2 mmol/l. All other electrolytes, including magnesium are within normal limits. You prescribe 20 mmol of potassium to be given in 100 ml saline over the next hour and arrange with the sister in charge of HDU to review him in an hour. When you review him, he is in sinus rhythm with a rate of 75 bpm, his CVP has risen to 6 mmHg and he has passed 30 ml of urine over the past 30 min. You change the fluid prescription to 1000 ml saline with 20 mmol KCl per litre 6-hourly and arrange to review the patient again later that evening.

### LEARNING POINTS
- use the CCrISP system of assessment to review all patients
- regular review of patients at risk will lead to early detection of potential problems
- correction of hypovolaemia, hypoxia and electrolyte disturbances is simple but is often very effective.

*DC cardioversion*
- should be considered early when very rapid rate or evidence of compromise, particularly for ventricular tachyarrythmias
- the patient must be anaesthetised
- less effective in cases of long-standing atrial arrhythmias
- appropriate help must be sought at an early stage.

*Pacing and surgical ablation*
The use of these treatments is beyond the scope of this manual. These should be used as a last resort under the guidance of a cardiologist.

## TABLE 6.6

### COMMON CAUSES OF ARRHYTHMIA

- Ischaemic heart disease
- Oxygen, fluid and electrolyte disturbances
- Drugs
- Rheumatic heart disease
- Cardiomyopathy
- Thyrotoxicosis

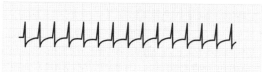

Figure 6.6 Supraventricular tachycardia.

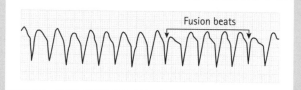

Figure 6.7 Ventricular tachycardia.

# VENTRICULAR TACHYARRYTHMIAS

## VENTRICULAR TACHYCARDIAS

Even the most common arrythmias (Table 6.6) may require cardiology input for safe and effective management. Ventricular tachycardias (VT) are potentially very serious and require prompt specialist referral. They should be distinguished from SVT by the appearance of the ECG (Figs. 6.6 and 6.7, Table 6.7). Cardioversion is often required for VT and this is particularly urgent if the patient has evidence of compromised cardiac output.

SVT may respond, although sometimes only temporarily, to intense vagal stimulus created by carotid sinus massage or the Valsalva manoeuvre. Otherwise, adenosine can be administered (0.05– 0.25 mg/kg). It has a powerful blocking effect on the AV node, thus slowing ventricular rate if the dysrhythmia is atrial in origin. It acts for only 15–20 seconds and is relatively safe in experienced hands. Its use should be avoided in the asthmatic and in the presence of dipyridamole, which greatly prolongs its action.

## TABLE 6.7

### DIFFERENTIATING SVT AND VT

| Chamber of origin | |
| --- | --- |
| *Supraventricular (SVT)* | *Ventricular (VT)* |
| QRS narrow complex | Often broad complex |
| Often no P waves | P waves dissociated rhythm |
| Usually regular | May be irregular |
| QRS right way up | QRS inverted |
| May respond to CSM | No response to CSM |
| Slowed with adenosine | No response to adenosine |

## VENTRICULAR ECTOPICS

Ventricular ectopics (VEs) may be unifocal (each ectopic will have the same shape) or multifocal (different shapes). The pulse will be irregular.

An ECG is the only certain way to distinguish this from other causes of irregular pulse. Their danger lies in the fact that an ectopic arising on the apex of a T wave may produce ventricular fibrillation. Clearly, the more ectopics there are, the greater is the probability of this happening. Treatment should be considered if the ratio of VE to normal QRS is greater than 1:6 or if multifocal. Lignocaine would be the treatment of choice.

## CLINICAL ASSOCIATION

VEs can occur in healthy people without evidence of any disease. The incidence is higher in older individuals. VEs also occur after MI, with electrolyte disturbance (*e.g.* hypokalaemia and hypomagnesaemia), in valvular heart disease, with cardiomyopathies, hypoxia and digitalis toxicity.

## COMMON TYPES OF ATRIAL TACHYCARDIA

### SINUS TACHYCARDIA

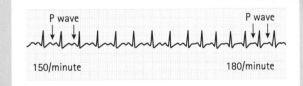

Figure 6.8 Sinus tachycardia.

- regular up to 160/min or so in young
- lesser maximum rate in older patients
- normal P wave and morphology
- gradual onset
- treat cause – hypovolaemia, anaemia, pulmonary embolism, sepsis, etc.

## PAROXYSMAL SUPRAVENTRICULAR TACHYCARDIA

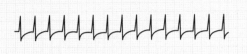

Figure 6.9 Paroxysmal SVT.

- any tachycardia originating in the AV node, atria or SA node
- P waves can be of abnormal shape and may or may not be seen
- QRS width usually normal (may be wide if associated bundle branch block)
- may be associated with ST depression, suggesting ischaemia
- regular 150–250/min
- abolished/slowed by carotid sinus massage and adenosine
- treatment: verapamil, digoxin, b-blockade (avoid in heart failure or with verapamil).

## ATRIAL FIBRILLATION

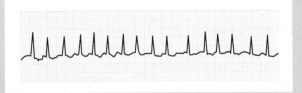

Figure 6.10 Atrial fibrillation.

- irregularly irregular; variable ventricular rate, often 100–180
- very common postoperatively in surgical patients
- associated with hypovolaemia, hypoxia and electrolyte disorders

- also associated with cardiopulmonary disease (*e.g.* ischaemic or rheumatic heart disease)
- no P waves, normal QRS.

## TREATMENT

The management of AF depends on the cause and effects. Many new cases occur after surgery, caused by hypovolaemia, hypoxia or electrolyte imbalance, particularly hypokalaemia and hypomagnesaemia. These episodes can be rapidly treated by correcting the causal factors alone. Identify and treat any underlying problems that would cause these predisposing factors to recur.

When new AF causes serious adverse signs (particularly hypotension, shock, chest pain, heart failure, decreased conscious level or marked tachycardia > 140), urgent treatment is needed either with DC cardioversion or intravenous amiodarone. Seek expert help immediately.

New AF, which does not cause serious adverse signs and which does not respond to the correction of the factors listed above, is usually treated with digoxin or amiodarone. Again, if problems persist or recur, or you are unsure, get expert help.

Long-standing AF can worsen after surgery if usual drugs have been omitted. This is unlikely to convert back to sinus rhythm without digoxin or amiodarone. Ultimately, anticoagulation may need to be considered.

- correct general causes as above, particularly hypoxia, hypovolaemia or hypomagnesaemia
- DC cardioversion – consider if acutely decompensated or following recent onset (more responsive)
- digoxin if reversal is not urgent
- amiodarone.

## ATRIAL FLUTTER

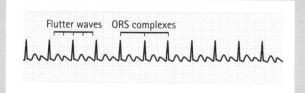

Figure 6.11 Atrial flutter.

- regular flutter P waves 300/min
- regular normal QRS, variable AV block
- usually associated with cardiac disease
- may respond to carotid massage, adenosine may reveal flutter waves
- atrial flutter and fibrillation may be present in the same patient
- treatment: cardioversion, digoxin, verapamil (care with digoxin).

### LEARNING POINT
Remember, in all the above cases, investigate the underlying cause!

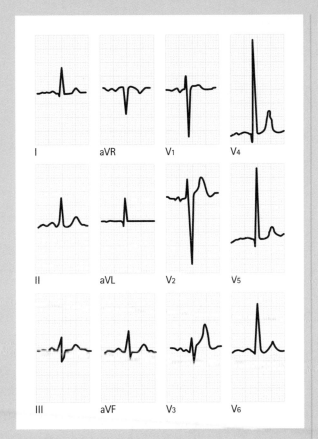

Figure 6.12 Left ventricular hypertrophy.

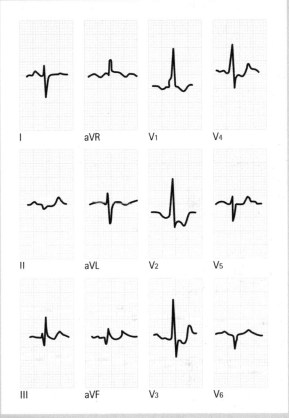

Figure 6.13 Right ventricular hypertrophy.

## LEFT VENTRICULAR HYPERTROPHY

A hypertrophied left ventricle has a greater influence on the electrical axis of the heart and causes left axis deviation. This gives the picture of tall R waves in I and aVL with S waves in III and aVF. Most noticeably, the increase in the left ventricular muscle mass also produces tall R waves in leads over the left ventricle (V4 to V6), and deep S waves in leads over the right ventricle (V1 to V3).

## CLINICAL ASSOCIATIONS

Conditions causing an increase in afterload or work on the left ventricle, for example, aortic valve disease, systemic hypertension.

## RIGHT VENTRICULAR HYPERTROPHY

When the electrical activity of the hypertrophied right ventricle predominates over the left, there is right axis deviation (leads I, II, III) with a tall R wave in V1 with deep S wave in V6. A tall pulmonary P wave suggests right atrial hypertrophy.

## CLINICAL ASSOCIATIONS
Conditions causing increased right ventricular afteload, for example, pulmonary hypertension, cor pulmonale, pulmonary stenosis.

## LEFT BUNDLE BRANCH BLOCK
Electrical activity in the left ventricle is delayed because conduction to it must take place via the right ventricle. The resultant delay in left ventricular depolarisation produces the 'M'-shaped QRS wave, typically in V5, V6, I and aVL, and a

'W'-shaped QRS in some of the reciprocal leads, typically leads III and aVF.

## RIGHT BUNDLE BRANCH BLOCK
Conversely, in right BBB, right ventricular depolarisation occurs via the left ventricle. In right BBB the 'M'-shaped QRS would typically be in leads V1, V2 and V3. Right BBB with left axis deviation suggests bi-fascicular block. This condition will often need pacing – seek help early!

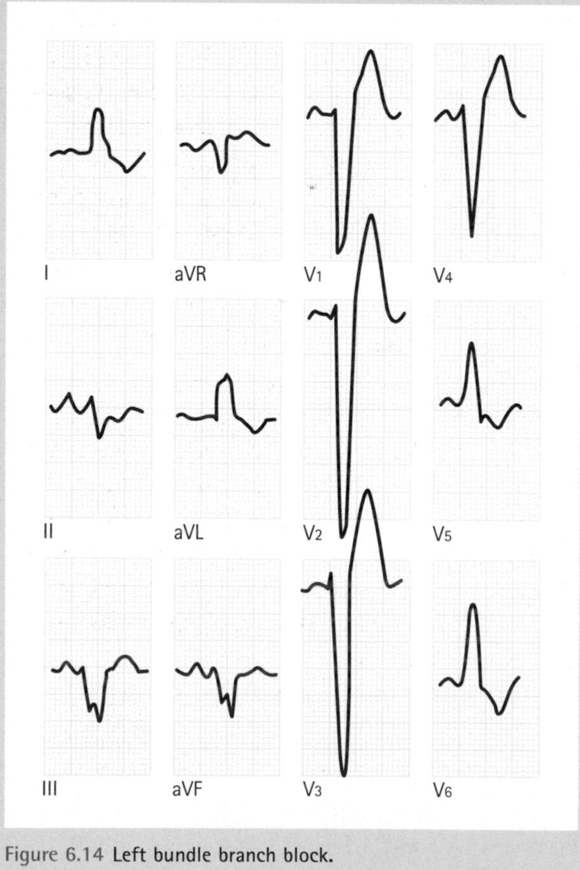

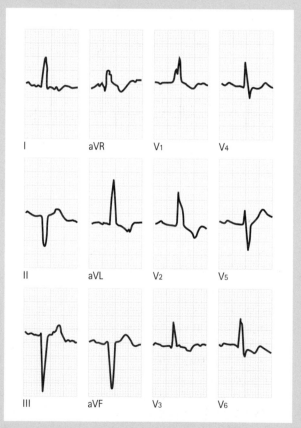

Figure 6.14 Left bundle branch block.

Figure 6.15 Right bundle branch block.

## CLINICAL ASSOCIATIONS

Coronary artery disease, valvular heart disease, ventricular hypertrophy and fibrosis, cardiomyopathies.

## BRADYARRYTHMIAS

Slow heart rates are problematic if associated with hypoperfusion or hypotension (Table 6.8). They are common in the elderly. The patient likely to get troublesome heart block (*e.g.* those with bi-fascicular block) should be detected pre-operatively and considered for elective pacing.

In the patient with symptomatic bradycardia, atropine (0.6–1.2 mg) may help but pacing may be needed. Isoprenaline infusion may be used under guidance of an intensivist or cardiologist. Discuss with your medical or ICU colleagues sooner rather than later!

## TABLE 6.8

### CONDITIONS ASSOCIATED WITH BRADYCARDIA

**Autonomic**
- Pain, especially visceral (may also be associated with tachycardia)
- Raised intracranial pressure
- Drugs: ß-blockers

**Non–autonomic**
- Myocardial infarction (particularly inferior MI)
- Gram-negative sepsis
- Hypoxia
- Drugs – digitalis toxicity
- Hypothyroidism
- Hypothermia.

## MYOCARDIAL INFARCTION

Ischaemic heart disease is very common, particularly in the elderly or in patients with peripheral or cerebro-vascular disease or diabetes mellitus. Peri-operative MI has a higher mortality than that occurring remote from operation. A recent MI (< 6 months) should preclude elective surgery since the incidence of peri-operative MI is increased within this period. ALL cardiac drugs should be continued up to and including the day of operation and recommenced at the earliest opportunity postoperatively. Peri-operative MI is often silent, though may present with shortness of breath, hypotension, evidence of decreased organ function (including confusion) secondary to cardiogenic shock, acute dysrhythmias, sudden pulmonary oedema or cardiac arrest. It should also enter the differential diagnosis of acute upper abdominal pain. A high index of suspicion is required particularly in high-risk groups.

The ECG may show typical changes of anterior, anterolateral or inferior MI with ST-segment elevation of > 1 mm in the relevant leads overlying the infarct (primary changes) and inversion in the leads opposite to it (reciprocal changes). T waves flatten and invert within hours to days of MI and Q waves develop over 1–2 days. Changes may be masked by a pre-existing left BBB and new BBB should make you suspicious. The ECG may be normal after an MI, certainly for the first hour or so. A normal ECG therefore does not exclude MI.

## PRACTICE POINT

*Recognition of patterns of ECG changes in MI:*
- Anterior infarct – primary changes V1, V2, V3, V4
- Inferior infarct – primary changes II, III, aVF
- Posterior infarct – isolated ST depression V1, V2

*Treatment*
- Oxygen, analgesia – refer and transfer to high-care area

Early treatment influences outcome significantly. If you suspect the presence of an MI then seek the advice of a physician urgently. In the meantime:
- check and correct the ABCs
- make the patient comfortable with a suitable opiate analgesic. Morphine (or diamorphine) is best, titrated to response intravenously (1–2 mg boluses every 2 minutes). Cyclizine (50 mg) or metoclopramide (10 mg) intravenously can be used to prevent or treat nausea
- give high flow oxygen to reduce hypoxia (monitor $SaO_2$)
- give glyceryl trinitrate (sublingual or spray) to reduce coronary artery spasm. Nitrates also have a synergistic effect with thrombolysis
- arrange appropriate investigations: (i) ECG (serial ECGs are required); and (ii) blood tests to exclude anaemia and electrolyte disturbances, and for troponin levels.

ECG changes of MI are localised to ischaemic or infarcted areas whereas generalised changes are seen in, for example, hyperkalaemia (peaked T waves) or pericarditis (ST elevation). The timing of changes is shown in Table 6.9.

### TABLE 6.9

#### TIME OF ECG CHANGES AFTER MI

| Change | Onset/duration |
| --- | --- |
| Peaked T waves | Seconds |
| ST changes (usually elevation) | Hours |
| Q waves | Hours–days |
| T wave inversion | Hours–days |

## ANTERIOR MYOCARDIAL INFARCTION

Raised ST segments in V1–V4.

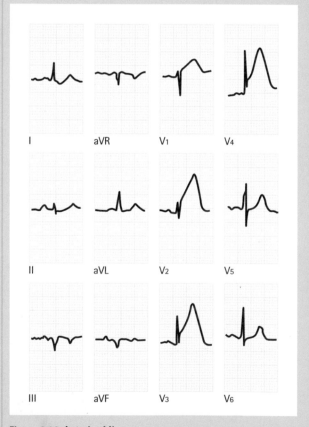

Figure 6.16 Anterior MI.

## INFERIOR MYOCARDIAL INFARCTION

Raised ST segments and Q waves can be seen in II, III, aVF leads (with reciprocal ST depression in leads I, aVL and V2–V4). Non-pathological Q waves can be present in leads II and III. Compare this with the example of the anterior infarction above.

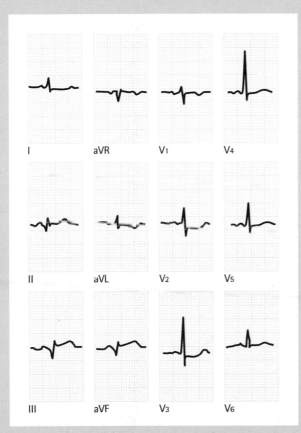

Figure 6.17 Inferior MI.

## ACUTE TREATMENT OF PROVEN MYOCARDIAL INFARCTION

THIS SHOULD BE INSTITUTED BY THE CARDIOLOGY TEAM BUT WILL REQUIRE CLOSE LIAISON WITH THE SURGICAL TEAM: THERE WILL NEED TO BE DISCUSSION REGARDING RISK OF BLEEDING VERSUS BENEFIT OF INTERVENTION, ANTICOAGULATION AND ANTI-PLATELET TREATMENT.

Acute treatment involves: (i) aspirin; (ii) clopidogrel; (iii) primary percutaneous intervention followed by anticoagulation with heparin or low molecular weight heparin; (iv) glycaemic control, particularly in diabetic patients (BM < 11 mmol/l); and (v) ß-blockers (providing there is no evidence of cardiac failure, bradycardia or hypotension, ß-blockers have been shown to improve survival).

If primary percutaneous intervention is not available, the fibrinolytics streptokinase or Alteplase (rTPA) can be used, particularly if there is persistent chest pain and gross ECG changes, though not in the immediate (< 2 weeks) post-operative period because of the risk of bleeding. Other contra-indications to fibrinolytics include:

- previous streptokinase treatment (further streptokinase contra-indicated – use rTPA)
- active peptic ulcer
- previous haemorrhagic stroke
- recent head injury, however minor
- prolonged traumatic CPR.

## ACUTE CORONARY SYNDROMES

'Acute coronary syndrome' is an increasingly used all-encompassing term that refers to a variety of myocardial conditions and includes acute MI (both Q wave and non-Q wave) and unstable angina. The full range of conditions included is listed in Table 6.10.

In most of these patients, the development of an acute coronary syndrome is due to rupture or erosion of an atherosclerotic plaque within the walls of a coronary artery, leading to thrombus formation. This is then followed by platelet aggregation and vasoconstriction of the associated vessels. Less commonly, an acute coronary syndrome is the result of emboli or coronary spasm. It is often impossible to distinguish between the different causes clinically.

### TABLE 6.10

#### THE ACUTE CORONARY SYNDROMES

**Acute myocardial infarction**
- Transmural myocardial infarction
- Q wave myocardial infarction
- ST elevation myocardial infarction (STEMI)

**Non-Q wave myocardial infarction**
- Sub-endocardial infarction
- Non-ST elevation myocardial infarction (non-STEMI)

**Unstable angina**

## TREATMENT STRATEGIES

AGAIN, THIS WILL NEED TO BE INSTITUTED BY THE CARDIOLOGY TEAM FOLLOWING SURGICAL DISCUSSION REGARDING RISK OF BLEEDING VERSUS BENEFIT OF ANTICOAGULATION AND ANTI-PLATELET TREATMENT.

- measure serial Troponin levels
- aspirin
- clopidogrel
- anticoagulation
- glycaemic control BM < 11 mmol/l
- ß-blockade

It is likely that patients with acute coronary syndromes will require further cardiology review and investigation prior to discharge.

## CONGESTIVE CARDIAC FAILURE

CCF is common in surgical critical care. It varies in severity from mild dyspnoea, which is easily treated, to cardiogenic shock. Demands on the heart are increased by surgical illness and this may unmask or worsen cardiac failure.

Cardiac function depends on preload, intrinsic myocardial function and afterload. This concept can be simplified in the following way. If the heart is thought of as a simple pump, the preload is analogous to the priming of the pump; it will only work well if it has something (and not too much) to pump. Ensuring adequate cardiac filling is essential. Any condition which disturbs 'pump filling' will affect preload and therefore cardiac function (Table 6.11a).

Intrinsic myocardial function is analogous to the function of the pump itself; if the pump fails in any way, it will not be able to cope with the demands made on it. Any condition that directly affects the function of cardiac muscle will affect intrinsic myocardial function (Table 6.11b). Afterload can be thought of as the work that is demanded of the pump to overcome the resistance to forward flow. If the resistance to flow is low, less work will be required of the pump; if it is high, the pump will have to work harder to produce an equal output. Conditions that alter circulatory resistance (systemic or pulmonary vascular resistance) or cause an obstruction to flow will affect afterload (Table 6.11c). Increases in afterload raise the cardiac oxygen demand, yet there is decreased supply to the sub-endocardial areas as the contracting muscle squeezes the sub-endocardial capillaries. If there is a simultaneous tachycardia the diastolic time interval is reduced and the coronary artery blood flow is reduced, decreasing myocardial oxygen delivery even more.

## TABLE 6.11

### CAUSES OF CARDIAC FAILURE IN SURGICAL CRITICAL CARE

**(a) Conditions affecting preload**

- hypovolaemia (bleeding, inadequate volume replacement, etc.)
- fluid overload
- pneumothorax/cardiac tamponade (b, c as well)

**(b) Conditions affecting intrinsic myocardial function**

- ischaemia
- infarction
- dysrhythmias
- chronic heart failure + 'operative stress'
- hypocalcaemia and other electrolyte disturbances
- myocardial depressant factors (*e.g.* in sepsis )
- pneumothorax/cardiac tamponade (see a, c as well)

**(c) Conditions affecting afterload**

- aortic/pulmonary valvular stenosis
- pulmonary embolism
- pneumothorax/cardiac tamponade (see a, b as well)
- aortic dissection

After surgery, a patient may develop CCF as a result of any of the conditions listed in Table 6.11. Sometimes, multiple factors apply in a single case and the range of specific disease processes that may produce these problems is wide. Most commonly, it is as a result of fluid overload. The cause of fluid overload may be obvious (*e.g.* giving blood or parenteral nutrition simultaneously with maintenance fluids to a patient with borderline cardiac function). Fluid balance can also become positive insidiously – perhaps as a result of several days of giving slightly too much maintenance fluid to a small, elderly patient, who may also have had routine diuretics omitted or developed AF.

The pathophysiolgy of CCF is such that patients enter a downward spiral of increasingly inefficient cardiac function. The physiological response to the failing heart (as it is to surgical pathology) is to increase catecholamine release in an attempt to stimulate cardiac output. Unfortunately, the failing heart has a 'flat Starling curve': one shifted down and to the right compared to the curve in Fig. 6.18. It is unable to respond and maintain cardiac output by increasing its stroke volume and tends to rely on an increase in rate. This is inefficient in that diastole is short, which reduces the time available for diastolic filling (affecting preload) and for perfusion of the coronary arteries leading to development of relative or absolute ischaemia (and further affecting intrinsic myocardial function).

Cardiogenic pulmonary oedema occurs with acute LVF or during an exacerbation of CCF. The patients usually have hypertension and ischaemic heart disease and are often elderly. They may develop symptoms as a result of MI or acute ischaemia precipitated by pain from non-cardiac sources. Sudden withdrawal of epidural analgesia may cause acute afterload increases in susceptible patients while increasing preload as the sympathetic block wears off. The commonest causes are iatrogenic fluid overload, dysrhythmia and MI. Patients become acutely dyspnoeic, orthopnoeic and tachypnoeic. They are tachycardic, sweaty, often hypertensive and a gallop rhythm may be present with a high JVP. They become hypoxic with increased work of breathing, which further aggravates myocardial ischaemia. Chest auscultation reveals crepitations basally with some wheeze (cardiac asthma) and, if very severe, pink, frothy sputum may be produced. The CXR may show fluid in the horizontal fissure, peribronchial cuffing, upper lobe diversion, perihilar 'bat's-wing' appearance and, rarely, Kerley B lines.

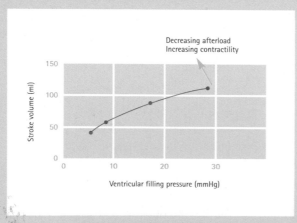

Figure 6.18 Cardiac function: Starling curve

## PRACTICE POINT

*Treatment follows ABC principles:*
- oxygen, sit the patient up, CPAP/BIPAP as soon as practicable
- diuretics and small doses of opiate intravenously to aid vasodilation
- reduce afterload as well as decreasing anxiety and dyspnoea
- if intravenous vasodilators/inotropes considered, transfer to high-care area.

## CASE SCENARIO 6.2

A 65-year-old woman with long-standing ischaemic heart disease had a right mastectomy 2 days ago. You are asked to see her on the third postoperative day because she has become acutely short of breath following an episode of severe central chest pain which lasted about 10 min but has since settled. When you arrive on the ward, the patient is obviously dyspnoeic and is unable to speak in complete sentences. She looks very unwell, and her skin feels cool and clammy. The staff nurse who is with her reports that her pulse rate is 110 bpm and her blood pressure is 170/95. You ask the nurse to give the patient high flow oxygen, using a mask with a reservoir bag. You examine the patient's chest and find that she has a respiratory rate of 28 breaths/min and fine crepitations up to the mid zones on both sides. It is difficult to hear her heart easily but you do not think you can hear any murmurs, although you think she has a gallop rhythm. Her blood pressure is now 140/90. You ask the nurse to help you sit the patient up and establish intravenous access. An examination of the patient's ward charts shows that she was progressing well until this episode. The case notes revealed that she is hypertensive, has occasional angina (about one attack every 2 weeks associated with exercise or cold weather) and usually takes bendrofluazide 2.5 mg and atenolol 50 mg each morning. From the prescription, it seems that she has not had these since her operation as she has felt nauseated due to the morphine PCA she has been using until recently. Although she seems slightly better with the oxygen and re-positioning, you decide to give her a dose of frusemide 40 mg i.v. You ask for an ECG to be obtained and order a CXR. The ECG shows a sinus tachycardia of 100 bpm but is otherwise unchanged from the one obtained pre-operatively. The CXR confirms pulmonary oedema. You arrange for the patient to be transferred to the high dependency ward where she can have continuous ECG, saturation and blood pressure monitoring and ask for her to be reviewed by the cardiology team. In the meantime, you arrange for routine blood tests and cardiac enzymes to be sent.

### LEARNING POINTS

- treat the ABCs first!
- give high flow oxygen to all patients during initial assessment
- many symptoms can be helped or relieved by repositioning of patients
- transfer to a higher level of care when closer monitoring is required
- seek expert help early.

The acute management of heart failure is as follows:

- assess and treat ABCs
- give oxygen and monitor $SaO_2$
- stop i.v. infusions (may be only temporary measure)
- drugs: consider diuretics (*e.g.* frusemide 80 mg i.v.), nitrates (patch, sublingual, buccal or i.v.), diamorphine 2.5–5 mg i.v. (but be sure of diagnosis – opiates can kill a patient with acute asthma or chronic bronchitis)
- 12-lead ECG
- treat any underlying cause such as dysrhythmia, pulmonary embolus or tamponade
- CVP monitoring
- early specialist referral.

Cardiogenic shock occurs when there is severe impairment of cardiac function with hypotension of less than 90 mmHg or 30 mmHg less than the patient's 'normal' systolic pressure is present. The patient may be tachycardic or bradycardic. Amongst the causes, the commonest is severe myocardial ischaemia or infarction. The cardiac output falls, systemic hypotension occurs and there is progressive fall in organ perfusion. Left ventricular end diastolic pressure rises and pulmonary venous pressure increases, which leads to pulmonary oedema formation. The patient becomes dyspnoeic and hypoxic and a downward spiral develops as low $SaO_2$ and low diastolic pressure further compromises myocardial perfusion. The acutely failing heart is exquisitely sensitive to too much or too little fluid. The patient normally has pulmonary oedema so increasing preload with i.v. fluid is often detrimental. Occasionally, the failing heart can have a high preload requirement and reducing preload by diuresis may worsen cardiac output. If the afterload is high, reducing it by using vasodilators may be beneficial but subsequent worsening hypotension may be detrimental to myocardial perfusion. Accurate individualised treatment requires the measurement of cardiac output, preload and afterload so invasive cardiac monitoring is required to optimise fluid loading, inotropic support and/or vasodilator therapy. Senior critical care input and monitoring is urgently needed.

## RISKS OF SURGERY

It is very important to be aware of the risks of surgery in the patient with ischaemic heart disease and, particularly, of the risk of re-infarction (Table 6.12). It should be evident that delaying surgery, if at all possible, will have a marked effect on the outcome.

### TABLE 6.12

RISK OF CARDIAC DISEASE IN NON-CARDIAC SURGERY

| Higher | Lower |
|---|---|
| Recent MI | MI > 6 months |
| Unstable angina | Stable angina |
| Severe aortic stenosis | Abnormal ECG |
| Decompensated heart failure | Compensated heart failure |
| Severe hypertension | Compensated valvular lesions |
| Cardiac arrhythmias | Cardiomegaly |

The risk of peri-operative MI is greater with abdominal and thoracic surgery and is related to the duration of operation. The chance of re-infarction has been estimated as:

- 60% if within 3 weeks of MI
- 27% if MI within 3 months of procedure
- 11% if MI within 3–6 months of procedure.

The presence of cardiac failure pre-operatively indicates a significant anaesthetic risk. Measurement of the ejection fraction can help quantitate this.

## HYPERTENSION

For a patient with chronic hypertension, avoid stopping long-term anti-hypertensive medication suddenly unless the patient is hypotensive. Remember to review the prescription chart of patients on cardiac drugs on a daily basis. As with almost all cardiac medication, it should be given on the morning of surgery and re-instituted as quickly as possible afterwards. Many anti-hypertensive drugs have side effects including hypokalaemia (diuretics), hyperkalaemia (ACE inhibitors) and impaired responses to hypovolaemia (vasodilators and ß-blockers).

Acute, life-threatening hypertension is rare. If the blood pressure is sustained at 220/120 or above with signs of organ dysfunction, involve cardiology immediately.

## PACEMAKERS

Patients who have pacemakers not infrequently require surgery. Pacemakers can vary between the simple fixed rate type (although these are rarely used now) to the complex demand type. They can be bipolar or unipolar, the casing acting as the return earth in the latter. It is vital to be aware that your patient has a pacemaker because the use of diathermy can inhibit the demand type, though this is less likely to cause problems with a standard fixed rate type. The important points are:

- any patient who has a pacemaker and requires surgery should have had a recent cardiology review to ensure the pacemaker is functioning optimally
- the diathermy earthing pad should be placed as far away from the pacemaker as possible (e g on the thigh or under the buttocks). Never place the pad on the back of the patient behind the pacemaker
- use short bursts of diathermy rather than long ones
- bipolar diathermy is safer than unipolar
- avoid using diathermy near the pacemaker if possible
- always monitor the ECG during any procedure.

Pacemaker types are classified using a 3 or 4 letter code. Classification is based on which chambers are paced, the response of the pacemaker to a sensed beat and programmability. Recognition of the codes and details of pacemaker function are beyond the scope of this manual and the CCrISP course. If you have any doubts or worries contact a cardiologist!

## SUMMARY

- the detection and treatment of early clinical signs can prevent major deterioration
- abnormal signs must be acted on quickly – patients deteriorate rapidly from cardiovascular problems
- normal clinical findings do not always exclude significant abnormality – further investigations and monitoring can help
- new and long-standing cardiac disorders occur frequently in surgical patients – be aware of common management strategies
- impaired perfusion, hypotension, end-organ dysfunction and poor response to treatment suggest severe problems
- patients with acute abnormalities of cardiovascular function should not be left without a clear management plan including appropriate treatment and a timely re-assessment
- higher levels of care are often required – either pre-emptively if the patient has long-standing problems pre-operatively, or in response to acute events
- seek specialist help (anaesthetic/cardiology/ICU) as appropriate at an early stage.

# 7

## Shock and haemorrhage

## OBJECTIVES

This chapter will help you to:

- define shock
- understand the various aetiologies of shock
- recognise the clinical features of a patient with shock
- initiate early treatment of the shocked patient
- based on the history, clinical condition and response to treatment, decide on an appropriate level of care.

This chapter aims to give a practical clinical overview rather than a detailed account of the pathophysiology of shock.

## DEFINITION

*Shock may be defined as acute circulatory failure, with inadequate tissue perfusion causing cellular hypoxia.*

Regardless of the underlying cause, shock is characterised by an acute alteration of the circulation in which inadequate perfusion leads to cellular damage, dysfunction and failure of major organ systems.

The clinical features of shock are so variable that they cannot be used to define the shocked state. Although the terms 'hypotension' and 'shock' are often taken to be synonymous, cellular perfusion may be inadequate despite a normal blood pressure. Perfusion describes blood flow but also implies the supply of substrates (including oxygen) and the removal of waste products. Use of the terminology 'inadequate tissue perfusion' rather than 'reduced perfusion' is important since blood flow and substrate supply may be increased in hypercatabolic states (*e.g.* trauma and sepsis) and yet inadequate for the demands of the tissues due to increased metabolism and failure to extract substrates from the circulation, especially in septic shock.

In the shocked state, the distribution of blood flow is important. While certain viscera preserve flow through autoregulation (*e.g.* heart, kidney), others cannot (*e.g.* skin, gut) and may be hypoperfused preferentially. Intestinal hypoperfusion may occur in the face of a normal pulse and blood pressure and, following a brief hypotensive episode, a prolonged period of intestinal hypoxia may occur, with generation of cytokines and the onset of systemic inflammation.

## LEARNING POINT

Patients may be in shock despite a normal systolic blood pressure.

## AETIOLOGY OF SHOCK

All patients with shock can be regarded as having generalised failure of the circulation. There are four principal categories of shock:
(i)  hypovolaemic;
(ii)  vasodilatory or apparent hypovolaemia;
(iii)  cardiogenic; and
(iv)  obstructive (see Fig. 7.1 and Table 7.1).
Within this classification, the various different causes of shock have common mechanisms with regard to the clinical manifestation of shock and these can be considered in terms of preload.

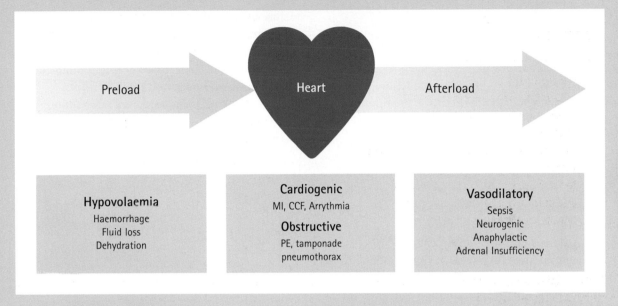

Figure 7.1 Classification of shock in relation to the effect on the circulation.

Rapid assessment of the patient may quickly suggest the cause of shock. Keeping this in mind, classification helps to avoid the risk of a given diagnosis being overlooked. Of course, the patient may have more than one factor contributing to the shock state: for example, a patient with abdominal sepsis where the primary problem is vasodilation but where hypovolaemia due to ileus also contributes.

| TABLE 7.1 | |
|---|---|
| **COMMON MECHANISMS OF SHOCK** | |
| Hypovolaemia | Blood or fluid loss |
| Cardiogenic | Pump failure |
| Septic | Early vasodilation |
| | Late pump failure |
| | Fluid loss from capillary leak |
| Neurogenic | Vasodilation |
| Anaphylactic | Vasodilation and pump failure |
| Obstructive | Prevents venous return to the heart |

## HYPOVOLAEMIC SHOCK

Stroke volume dictates cardiac output, and is directly linked to ventricular filling pressure by the Starling curve (Fig. 7.2). Remember that the curve can be shifted up and to the left by inotropes and sympathetic stimulation. It is important to consider the Starling curve when thinking about the clinical manifestation of shock, but also rationale and response to treatment. Hypovolaemia is the commonest cause of shock in the surgical patient. The low cardiac output is a direct reflection of reduced venous return (preload). It may result from any of the following causes:

- haemorrhage is a common cause of hypovolaemia. Its effects vary with the duration and severity of blood loss, the patient's age and myocardial condition, and the speed and adequacy of resuscitation. It can be usefully classified, in terms of assessment and guiding treatment, by the degree of blood loss into four stages: stage 1, < 500 ml; stage 2, 500–1000 ml; stage 3, 1000–2000 ml; and stage 4, > 2000 ml
- loss of gastrointestinal fluid may result from vomiting and diarrhoea, from fistulae, and from sequestration of fluid in the bowel lumen in intestinal obstruction
- trauma and infection increase capillary permeability with local sequestration of fluid and oedema. In addition to causing hypovolaemia, trauma and infection may lead to sepsis
- burns lead to direct loss of fluid from the burned surface and tissue fluid sequestration
- renal loss of water and electrolytes (*e.g.* in sodium-losing chronic nephritis, diabetic ketosis or Addisonian crisis) is an occasional cause of shock
- frequently, iatrogenic surgical factors contribute to hypovolaemia (*e.g.* poor fluid prescription, slow or tissued intravenous infusion, inappropriate use of diuretics, mechanical bowel preparation, fasting prior to anaesthesia, and insensible fluid losses during prolonged operations and on going fluid loss from dissected areas for some hours after surgery).

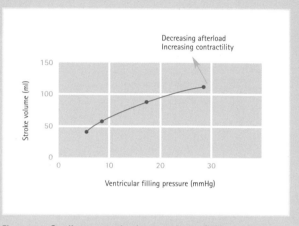

Figure 7.2 Starling curve plotting ventricular filling pressure (venous return) against stroke volume (cardiac output). The curve is shifted up and to the left by sympathetic stimulation or inotropic agents.

## CARDIOGENIC SHOCK

Primary impairment of cardiac function may result from myocardial infarction or ischaemia, acute arrhythmias, acute cardiomyopathy, acute valvular lesions (caused by aortic dissection or trauma), and myocardial contusion.

## OBSTRUCTIVE SHOCK

Secondary impairment to cardiac function can result from obstruction to cardiac output. Causes include cardiac tamponade producing constriction of the heart, pressure on the heart from a tension pneumothorax or major pulmonary embolism with obstruction to right ventricular outflow.

In all shock states, myocardial performance is affected adversely by reduced coronary arterial perfusion and, in some cases, by circulating myocardial depressant substances (particularly in septic shock).

## NEUROGENIC FACTORS

True neurogenic shock follows spinal transection or brain-stem injury with loss of sympathetic outflow beneath the level of injury and consequent vasodilation. The rapid increase in size of the vascular bed, including venous capacitance vessels, leads to reduced venous return and reduced cardiac output. There is often a relative bradycardia. An analogous condition may be seen during epidural analgesia, although in this case, the block is seldom high enough to cause a bradycardia.

## ANAPHYLAXIS

Anaphylactic reactions are mediated by IgE antibodies causing massive degranulation of mast cells in sensitised individuals. Activation of mast cells releases histamine and serotonin and, with systemic kinin activation, this leads to rapid vasodilation, a fall in systemic vascular resistance (SVR), hypotension, severe bronchospasm with hypoxia and hypercarbia. In contrast to sepsis, the fall in SVR is so sudden and profound that blood pressure falls markedly. Prompt treatment with oxygen, fluids, adrenaline, hydrocortisone and an antihistamine is required plus avoidance of the trigger substance.

## ENDOCRINE FACTORS

Although adrenal failure is in itself a potent cause of shock due to the sudden withdrawal of circulating cortisol and aldosterone, the role of the adrenal cortex in the production of shock by other causes is debatable. Acute adrenal failure may occur in severe meningococcal sepsis (Waterhouse–Friedrichsen syndrome). Adrenal insufficiency (often subacute) is also seen in patients in whom necessary peri-operative steroid cover has been omitted.

## SEPTIC SHOCK

Sepsis and septic shock are complex and are covered in more detail elsewhere. In septic shock, the patient becomes hypotensive and the tissues are inadequately perfused as a result of organisms, toxins or inflammatory mediators. Common sources include the abdomen, chest, soft tissues, wounds, urine and intravascular lines (central or peripheral) or other medical implants.

## CASE SCENARIO 7.1

You receive a trauma team call to the emergency department – the paramedics have radioed that they will be arriving in 4 min with a 34-year-old patient who has a BP of 80 systolic and a stab wound to the back between the shoulder blades.

WHAT FORM OF SHOCK MIGHT THIS PATIENT BE SUFFERING FROM?
Haemorrhagic shock? 'Pump failure' due to pericardial tamponade? 'Pump failure' due to tension pneumothorax? Neurogenic shock due to spinal cord transection? All are possible!

WHAT ACTION MAY BE NECESSARY?
This depends on the cause, but immediate attention to the ABCs with administration of oxygen and fluids, diagnosis and definitive treatment are the mainstays of treatment.

# CLINICAL FEATURES OF SHOCK

## ASSESSMENT

It is essential that you follow the systematic approach of the CCrISP algorithm when assessing the potentially shocked patient. Perform the immediate assessment with simultaneous resuscitation, followed by a full patient assessment, including chart review, history, examination and investigations. For a patient on a surgical ward, it is also important to speak to the medical and nursing staff, and note the results of recent investigations and procedures.

### IMPORTANT FEATURES TO NOTE

- is there an obvious cause which requires immediate treatment?
- does the age or previous history of a patient suggest a possible myocardial component?
- has the patient recently received medication which may have an effect on the cardiovascular or respiratory systems?
- does the fluid balance chart of the patient show a gradually deteriorating urine output or likelihood of a significantly abnormal fluid balance? Remember that trends in the charted observations may be more important than absolute values and that patients with hypovolaemic shock may have a normal systolic blood pressure
- does the patient have a temperature, high white cell count or a history of an operative procedure which may make sepsis a more likely diagnosis?

The majority of patients with shock have a low cardiac output; an exception is septic shock where the cardiac output may be increased. The classical appearance of a patient with low-output shock is that seen after haemorrhage. The features are partly due to loss of circulating volume and tissue perfusion, and partly to intense sympathetic stimulation. Early diagnosis of shock depends on recognition of the signs of decreased tissue perfusion, particularly of the skin, kidneys and brain.

Signs of decreased tissue perfusion are summarised in Table 7.2. These are accompanied by varying degrees of tachycardia, hypotension and tachypnoea proportional to the severity of the shock. Increased respiratory rate is frequently seen before significant tachycardia, but marked tachypnoea is an important sign of impending deterioration. Confusion and coma are late signs of marked cerebral hypoperfusion, and blood pressure is often maintained until severe shock.

### TABLE 7.2

#### SIGNS OF DECREASED TISSUE PERFUSION

- Cool peripheries
- Poor filling of peripheral veins
- Increased respiratory rate
- Increased core–peripheral temperature gradient
- Capillary refill time prolonged (> 2 s)
- Poor signal on pulse oximeter
- Poor urine output (< 0.5 ml/kg body weight/h)
- Restlessness or decreased conscious level
- Metabolic acidosis or elevated lactate levels

In haemorrhagic shock, decreased venous return to the heart results in a low right atrial pressure, low right ventricular end diastolic volume and reduced right heart output. This usually reduces the left atrial and ventricular end diastolic volumes and stroke volume falls. Since cardiac output (CO) = heart rate (HR) x stroke volume (SV), for a fixed SV, an increase in HR is the first compensatory measure available. The only way the body has to increase the SV acutely is to decrease the amount of blood contained in the resistance and capacitance vessels by vasoconstriction, squeezing the periphery to return more blood to the heart. This gives the appearance of the cold shut down peripheries. The patient's response to hypovolaemia may be modified in the elderly, in ischaemic heart disease, in patients on ß-blockers, trained athletes and young adults

The effect of haemorrhage on blood pressure is particularly variable. It depends on the duration and magnitude of blood loss, the patient's age and cardiovascular status, and the speed and adequacy of resuscitation. Initially, the systemic blood pressure is maintained, and may actually increase, particularly in young patients. The pulse pressure may drop (difference between systolic and diastolic pressure) as a result of peripheral vasoconstriction but this is a subtle sign. Up to 25% (or even 30%) of circulating volume can be lost without affecting systolic pressure because of the intense vasoconstriction and, to a lesser extent, the shift of fluid from interstitial to intravascular space. A modest further loss (to 35–40% deficit) can precipitate calamitous collapse, perhaps with bradycardia rather than the expected tachycardia.

## PRACTICE POINT

*Systolic blood pressure may be normal in the presence of significant loss of circulating volume.*

## SPECIFIC FEATURES OF CARDIOGENIC SHOCK

Cardiogenic shock is inadequate tissue perfusion resulting directly from myocardial dysfunction. Common causes in surgical patients include myocardial infarction, acute arrhythmias, post-cardiac surgery myocardial 'stunning' and cardiac contusions from trauma. The clinical features are similar to hypovolaemic shock. Although there is no primary loss of circulating volume, cardiac output falls and catecholamine-induced vasoconstriction produces cool clammy peripheries, reduced capillary return, reduced urine output and reduced level of consciousness. The picture is modified, however, by elevation of cardiac filling pressure leading to elevation of the central or jugular venous pressure and pulmonary oedema, but low arterial pressure.

A careful history and examination of the chest, heart sounds (there may be a gallop rhythm or associated murmur), neck veins together with assessment of a chest radiograph and ECG should prevent the possibility of cardiogenic shock being overlooked in a surgical patient. Echocardiography may be valuable.

## SPECIFIC FEATURES OF OBSTRUCTIVE SHOCK

Cardiac tamponade, tension pneumothorax and pulmonary embolism are the principal causes of obstructive shock. Through a variety of mechanisms, each restricts the work of the heart, leading to a drop in the CI. Typically, the JVP can be elevated in each and assessment of the JVP should be routine. Tamponade and tension pneumothorax need prompt intervention to relieve the pressure on the heart, but all can respond temporarily to intravenous fluids and oxygen.

## SPECIFIC FEATURES OF SEPTIC SHOCK

Sepsis is dealt with and defined elsewhere in this book and further comments here are limited to the making of a diagnosis. Clearly, haemodynamic instability and pyrexia 5–7 days after a colonic resection with anastomosis should be treated with suspicion but, in general, the early features of sepsis (Table 7.3) are subtle, diagnosis is difficult and a high index of suspicion is essential. The patient may look remarkably well, largely due to pink, well-perfused extremities. As already stressed, clues may be obtained from the history or the patient's charts; in postoperative patients, blood gas measurements can aid early diagnosis.

### PRACTICE POINT

*A grave error is for inexperienced personnel to treat restlessness (due to hypoxia and hypovolaemia) with sedation rather than appropriate resuscitation.*

### TABLE 7.3

#### CLINICAL FEATURES OF SEPSIS

| Early | Late |
| --- | --- |
| Restlessness and slight confusion | Decreased conscious level |
| Tachypnoea | Tachypnoea |
| Tachycardia | Tachycardia |
| Low SVR | |
| High cardiac output | Low cardiac output |
| Systolic BP normal or slightly decreased | Systolic BP less than 80 mmHg |
| Oliguria | Oliguria |
| Metabolic acidosis, elevated blood lactate | Metabolic acidosis, elevated blood lactate |
| Warm, dry, suffused extremities | Cold extremities |

In septic shock, an early effect of the mediators is to cause a fall in SVR due to vasodilation. The decrease in SVR reduces the afterload on the heart and leads to a reflex increase in cardiac output, provided the patient has a healthy myocardium and adequate volume state. Thus, in early sepsis, blood pressure may be well maintained, and often the patient is pink with flushed peripheries and maybe a low diastolic pressure. This is in contrast to cardiogenic or pure hypovolaemic shock where the SVR rises in response to the drop in cardiac output.

In the later stages, or if the patient is already hypovolaemic, the heart may be unable to maintain an adequate output in the face of a falling SVR, so that blood pressure falls (BP = CO x SVR). The patient may then become almost indistinguishable from someone suffering from hypovolaemic shock. Hence, the patient may be hypothermic or hyperthermic depending on the phase. As the septic process progresses, fluid loss due to increased capillary permeability may also contribute to hypotension and, in addition, myocardial depressant factors reduce cardiac function directly. Initially, the patient requires oxygen and fluids but it is vital that cultures are taken and the source is identified and treated.

## PRINCIPLES OF MONITORING AND MANAGEMENT

Restoration of adequate perfusion at the cellular level is the essential aim of treatment. In practice, the initial resuscitation of patients with any form of shock is influenced more by the nature of the associated physiological disturbances than by the specific underlying cause. On the other hand, the ultimate success of treatment depends largely on detection and elimination of the underlying cause (*e.g.* arrest of bleeding or drainage of a source of sepsis).

---

### PRACTICE POINT

*In monitoring and management, the essential principles are:*
- *resuscitate*
- *diagnose*
- *treat underlying cause.*

---

The mainstays of early treatment are infusion of fluid and oxygen administration with the aim of improving cardiac output and oxygen transport. If cardiogenic and obstructive forms of shock can be excluded, all patients with shock can be initially treated with fluid administration (initial bolus 10 ml/kg body weight crystalloid if normotensive, 20 ml/kg body weight if hypotensive). Oxygen should initially be given in high concentration (12–15 l/min) until blood gas analysis or saturation measurements are available.

Occasionally, you will encounter a patient with major haemorrhage who requires operative resuscitation. You will find it very difficult to resuscitate a patient with major haemorrhage; prolonged attempts are futile and merely lead to coagulopathy, hypothermia and death. Exsanguinating patients need immediate definitive treatment – usually by surgery.

As stressed above, it is the indices of tissue perfusion which are most useful in the early management of hypovolaemia. One should not be misled into thinking that a patient is well perfused simply because the blood pressure and heart rate are normal. On the other hand, a lucid patient with rapid capillary refill, warm dry skin, and a good urine output is unlikely to have significant hypovolaemia.

### MONITORING AND INSTRUMENTATION

Successful clinical monitoring depends on the frequent measurement of simple haemodynamic indices and assessment of tissue perfusion, as just outlined. The following guidelines apply to all forms of shock.

*Venous access*

Good venous access must be obtained early by inserting at least two large-bore (16G) peripheral cannulae. Access is normally obtained in the antecubital fossa or via the cephalic vein at the wrist. If vasoconstriction makes it difficult to gain access, a 'cut-down' can be performed in the antecubital fossa or on the long saphenous vein in front of the medial malleolus. In profoundly shocked patients, it may be necessary to obtain the initial access by cannulating the femoral vein percutaneously in the groin. Draw blood for urgent cross-matching, haematology and biochemistry.

*Bladder catheterisation*

A bladder catheter is inserted transurethrally unless there is a possibility of urethral injury (as in severe pelvic fractures), or when dealing with young children. Under these circumstances, a suprapubic catheter is inserted once the bladder has filled, under ultrasound control. The urinary catheter is attached to a graduated collecting device (urimeter) so that output can be measured hourly.

*Electrocardiogram (ECG) monitoring*

ECG monitoring will detect arrhythmias and myocardial ischaemia. It is indicated particularly in primary cardiogenic shock, myocardial dysfunction secondary to ischaemia, direct thoracic injury, and sepsis. Arrhythmias are more likely when there is electrolyte or acid–base disturbance.

*Pulse oximetry*

A pulse oximeter attached to a finger or ear lobe allows transcutaneous estimation of oxygen saturation of haemoglobin. The accuracy of such peripheral probes depends on good peripheral perfusion. However, in poorly perfused patients, good equipment gives a visual or audible warning of a poor signal, so providing a useful index of both oxygen transport and tissue perfusion.

*Central venous catheterisation*

A catheter can be inserted percutaneously via the internal jugular or subclavian veins so that it lies in the superior vena cava, thus allowing measurement of CVP. In the initial resuscitation of an overtly hypovolaemic patient, time must not be wasted inserting a central venous catheter. The small bore and length of the catheter usually prevent rapid infusion, while inadvertent damage to the apical pleura during insertion may lead to a pneumothorax, a potentially fatal complication in a patient who is not resuscitated. Furthermore, central lines are no longer the remit of the junior surgeon and should be placed by anaesthetists in a controlled environment with the use of ultrasound guidance. However, following the initial administration of fluid and oxygen, measurement of CVP can be useful, particularly in severe shock and if there is clinical uncertainty.

In a shocked patient, a low (< 5 mmHg) or even negative CVP indicates the need for more fluid. At the other extreme, a very high CVP (> 20 mmHg) may indicate cardiac failure and the need for diuretics, vasodilators or inotropic agents, or an obstructive cause. In practice, static measurement of CVP can mislead. For example, a young patient may have an apparently normal CVP (say 10 mmHg) as a result of vasoconstriction. A 'fluid challenge' can resolve doubt. This is performed by measuring CVP before and after the administration of a small fluid bolus (100–200 ml). If the CVP does not rise, further fluid can be given safely; a significant rise in CVP suggests myocardial failure or dysfunction and avoids inadvertent overtransfusion (Fig. 7.3).

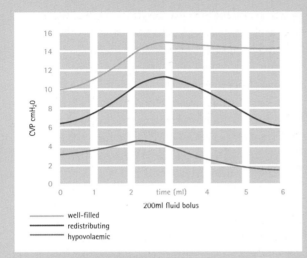

Figure 7.3 CVP response to a 200-ml bolus in different clinical situations.

## CORE AND PERIPHERAL TEMPERATURE MEASUREMENT

Using one's own hand to assess skin temperature is useful in shocked patients. If thermistors are used to measure core and peripheral temperatures, the core–peripheral gradient provides a useful index of skin perfusion. Core temperature measurement also detects hypothermia, as in trauma patients who have been exposed to a cold environment, particularly following water immersion.

## FLUID ADMINISTRATION

In most cases, the type of fluid lost in shock has little influence on the choice of fluid for initial replacement. Successful initial resuscitation depends more on the rapidity and adequacy of fluid replacement than on the choice of regimen. Initial fluid management consists of boluses of warmed crystalloid (10–20 ml/kg body weight). However, red cell concentrates may be required at an early stage, particularly amongst the injured

or patients who are bleeding. Subsequent administration depends on monitoring the response to treatment and all shocked patients need careful and repeated assessments (Table 7.4).

## TABLE 7.4

### CONTINUING ASSESSMENT OF THE SHOCKED PATIENT

Monitor clinical appearance, noting restlessness and confusion (cerebral hypoxia), respiratory rate and state of the peripheral circulation

Monitor pulse rate, systemic blood pressure, hourly urine output and CVP

Gain valuable additional information by monitoring or periodically checking:
- blood urea and electrolyte concentrations
- haemoglobin concentration, white cell count and haematocrit
- ABGs
- blood lactate level
- pulse oximetry
- core and peripheral temperature
- CI

Remember to send appropriate samples for bacteriological examination (*e.g.* blood, urine, sputum, drain fluids) when sepsis is suspected, and cardiac monitoring/serial ECGs in cardiogenic shock

Most importantly, diagnose and treat the underlying cause

Infusion of large volumes of fluid (of any type, including red cell concentrates) can cause dilution of clotting factors (factors II, V, VII, IX, X and platelets). The resulting coagulopathy may need correction by transfusion of fresh frozen plasma, platelets and cryoprecipitate. This should be done selectively rather than routinely but a watch must be kept for evidence of coagulopathy. Hospitals usually have guidelines for the use of clotting factors and you should be aware of these.

Considerable degrees of coagulopathy can be simply observed and monitored in the absence of active bleeding, but clotting factors are required early if the patient is bleeding or surgery is likely. Hypothermia also contributes to a bleeding diathesis by causing platelet dysfunction. Ensure that resuscitation fluids are warmed, particularly when massive transfusion is needed.

*Colloid or crystalloid?*
Synthetic colloids increase circulating volume to a greater degree in the short term per volume infused, but most are redistributed within a few hours in a similar manner to saline. All carry a risk of side effects, notably anaphylaxis and coagulopathy. You should recall to which fluid compartment each fluid type is distributed and also the mechanisms whereby circulating volume is supported by the extracellular and intracellular compartments during hypovolaemic states.

The debate over colloid or crystalloid is well documented. Some of the salient points are:
- in most situations, both types of fluid are able to replenish blood volume if given in sufficient quantity
- to replace a given amount of blood loss, the volume of crystalloid is approximately three times that of colloid

- when crystalloid resuscitation is used, there is a greater weight gain and probably more oedema than when colloid is used
- there is no fixed relationship between serum albumin concentration and colloid osmotic pressure until serum albumin falls below 15 g/l
- in septic shock with increased capillary permeability, both colloids and crystalloids pass across the vascular basement membrane
- colloid can interfere with coagulation under some circumstances
- many experienced practitioners would limit the volume of colloid used during resuscitation to < 50% of non-blood fluid or 1–1.5 l, whichever is less.

More importantly, the principal changes in practice that occur with experience are the early identification and rapid treatment of hypovolaemic states, a prompt utilisation of blood when haemorrhage is occurring and, most importantly, the surgical treatment of any underlying cause, particularly haemorrhage.

## ASSESSMENT OF RESPONSE
One of the most important steps in the management of the shocked patient is the assessment of the response to treatment. For every exsanguination, you will meet many more patients who become critically ill with shock in a less dramatic, but no less important manner. During resuscitation and no more than every 30 minutes or so, you should re-assess the patient's progress. If the signs are not improving, you need to change your plan of action (Table 7.5). The aim is to detect those patients you have initially misjudged or those who are temporary responders. These patients are common and it can be difficult to assess the need for surgery. Involve senior help if you are in doubt.

## CASE SCENARIO 7.2

You are called to see a 68-year-old man on the surgical ward. He is 5 days postoperative following a difficult anterior resection for a colonic tumour. He weighs 125 kg, has NIDDM, and a history of hypertension. He has been spiking a temperature for the last 48 h but has remained reasonably well until now. It is 8 p.m., and the nurses on the ward are concerned because he has become cold, clammy and restless. You follow the CCrISP protocol and establish that the airway is clear. His $SaO_2$ is 92%, respiratory rate 28 per min, pulse 110 and the urine output has been 20 ml over the last hour. He is restless but co-operative.

### WHAT FORM OF SHOCK MIGHT THIS MAN HAVE AND WHAT WOULD YOU DO?

Hypovolaemic/haemorrhagic shock? Cardiogenic shock? Septic shock? Obstructive shock? All are possible and there may be more than one pathology here. He has been spiking a temperature, so sepsis is possible. This might also have led to a secondary haemorrhage. He has risk factors for cardiac disease, and myocardial infarction or acute arrhythmia, possibly related to sepsis, is quite possible. He may also have had a pulmonary embolism causing obstructive shock. Following the CCrISP protocol, you should quickly be able to ascertain which type of shock is most likely. You institute high flow oxygen, gain intravenous access and send blood samples including cross-match and cultures. The BP is 115/60 which you note from chart review has dropped. His urine output has also tailed off. Abdominal examination is difficult but feels tense. There is no acute change on ECG.

### HOW WOULD YOU FURTHER MANAGE THIS SITUATION?

This man is clearly shocked and needs simultaneous assessment and resuscitation. The response to a fluid challenge while you wait for available results will give you a much better idea of the problem. You give a fluid challenge of 20 ml/kg body weight and re-assess. His BP initially rises to 140/80, but then drops again and he remains restless and tachycardic. On a blood gas, his Hb is 7 g/dl, and he has a metabolic acidosis with lactate of 5.

### WHAT ACTION MAY BE NECESSARY?

The most likely cause here is secondary haemorrhage, possibly secondary to intra-abdominal sepsis. He is a temporary responder and needs further intervention (probably surgery) to deal with the cause. You must seek help at this stage! As a bare minimum, he needs a higher level of care, with invasive monitoring and further aggressive resuscitation.

### LEARNING POINTS

- There may be more than one cause of shock — the CCrISP system will help you to decide.
- Shock may not be amenable to resuscitation alone — surgery may be required to stop the bleeding or deal with the cause.
- Some surgical patients are difficult to assess — if you are not sure, or a patient fails to respond to simple resuscitative measures, get help early.

## TABLE 7.5

### RESPONSES TO TREATMENT OF SHOCK

- No response, *e.g.* exsanguination
- Temporary response, *e.g.* continuing slow but steady postoperative haemorrhage
- Full response, *e.g.* simple sepsis caused by repeat urinary catheterisation which responds to resuscitation and antibiotics

## REFRACTORY SHOCK

If hypovolaemic shock proves refractory to fluid replacement and oxygen administration, the factors shown in Table 7.6 may be responsible.

## TABLE 7.6

### REFRACTORY SHOCK

- Underestimation of the degree of hypovolaemia
- Failure to arrest haemorrhage
- Presence of cardiac tamponade or tension pneumothorax
- Underlying sepsis
- Secondary cardiovascular effects due to delay in instituting treatment
- Further action is necessary!

*Algorithm of cardiovascular monitoring/support*

An algorithm of cardiovascular monitoring/support is given in Table 7.7. Many surgical patients become hypovolaemic and present with oliguria, hypotension, tachycardia, hypoxia or acidosis in isolation or almost any combination. Many do not develop a full picture of shock but require prompt treatment just the same. Most are simply treated with conventional measures including adequate fluid replacement (and other necessary treatments). You need to have a method of management clear in your mind. You should review them later to ensure that normal function has definitely been re-established. Patients who need anything more than simple correction of minor-to-modest fluid deficit should be managed in a high-dependency environment.

## TABLE 7.7

### ALGORITHM OF CARDIOVASCULAR MONITORING/SUPPORT

**1. Establish and maintain normovolaemia**
- Assess with CCrISP system
- Give reasonable intravenous fluid challenge (10–20 ml/kg crystalloid initially, see text)
- Treat any underlying cause (blood loss, sepsis, etc.)
- Determine recent fluid balance

**2. Assess response**
- Clinically (perfusion, BP, urine output, JVP, pulse)
- By simple investigations (repeat FBC, pulse oximetry, pH, BE)
- *Improving*, adjust fluid regimen, treat underlying cause, plan to review shortly
- *Deteriorating*, resuscitate and involve expert help directly
- *No progress*, re-assess – different diagnosis, treat and seek help; still hypovolaemic, continue fluids and find/treat cause
- *Not sure if normovolaemic*, insert CVP and seek higher level of care

**3. CVP**
- *Inadequate*, establish normovolaemia
- *Adequate* c > 8 cmH$_2$O), but inadequate circulation: re-assess cause (and treat as necessary); consider inotrope in higher level of care; no/poor response, seek help directly
- *High* c > 15 cmH$_2$O), and patient exhibits signs of cardiac failure: simple LVF, treat; suspect cardiogenic shock, call for help

**4. Invasive monitoring and inotrope treatment**
- Transfer to ICU

Remember to treat any underlying pathology, particularly haemorrhage (which often needs surgery), in addition to giving intravenous fluids and oxygen.

Patients who have incipient failure of more than one system need the help of an intensivist directly and, in any event, you should have a very low threshold for involving help and informing your consultant. All these patients should be receiving monitored oxygen therapy.

Young and fit patients tolerate rapid infusion well and CVP insertion is indicated when there is doubt about progress, adequacy of filling or likely tolerance of the administered fluid.

Patients who continue with inadequate cardiovascular function and in whom good cardiovascular filling has been confirmed by CVP measurement may require inotropic support. In these cases senior help should be mandatory and patients should be treated in a critical care environment. In some units, local protocols may allow administration of a single inotrope outside the intensive care unit, but these should be administered cautiously with a low threshold for transfer to the (ICU), with whom the case should already have been discussed.

*Metabolic monitoring in refractory shock*
Urea and electrolyte levels are required to establish a baseline and monitor progress. Arterial pH and blood gas measurements are essential to assess hypoxia, hypercapnia and acid–base balance. Blood lactate levels are a good index of cellular hypoxia and hepatic function.

Metabolic acidosis associated with inadequate perfusion will correct rapidly once cardiac output is improved; indeed, its disappearance is a marker of adequate resuscitation. It is rarely necessary to give bicarbonate.

Respiratory acidosis with an increase in arterial $PaCO_2$ usually indicates the need for endotracheal intubation and assisted ventilation.

*Higher levels of care*
Shock is an immediate life-threatening condition and demands treatment as such. The ability of the cardiovascular system to compensate has been discussed and shock reflects the state which is reached once decompensation is occurring. While uncomplicated hypovolaemia can often be managed satisfactorily without intensive care facilities, patients with severe trauma, sepsis, cardiogenic shock or shock complicated by secondary myocardial dysfunction will all benefit from the monitoring and support available in an ICU.

Consideration should be given to early ICU admission for patients with significant co-morbidity, since ICU can then play a prophylactic role. Similarly, patients who fail to respond quickly and completely should be discussed with ICU and a surgical consultant. Assessment and monitoring of the cardiovascular system is detailed elsewhere. The basis of ICU care is the same as outlined previously with attention to fluid administration, oxygenation and definitive treatment.

Based on the underlying cause of shock and measurement of cardiovascular parameters (particularly the confirmation of an adequate circulatory volume), some patients require inotropic support. The selection of an inotropic agent is based on the cardiovascular effects of the drug and the underlying pathophysiology. The cardiovascular effects of many agents can be predicted from a knowledge of their particular effect on adrenergic receptors (see Chapter 8).

## SUMMARY

*Definition*
- acute circulatory failure, with inadequate tissue perfusion causing
- cellular hypoxia.

*Diagnosis*
- assess perfusion and not simply blood pressure
- identify the different common patterns.

*Treatment*
- restore perfusion
- common initial approach with oxygen and fluids except for cardiogenic
- treat underlying cause
- determine appropriate level of care.

# 8

## Cardiovascular monitoring and support

## OBJECTIVES

This chapter will help you to:

- understand the indications for cardiovascular monitoring and support
- be familiar with the methods used
- understand how drug and fluid therapy may be used to manipulate cardiovascular function.

## INTRODUCTION

Maintaining adequate tissue perfusion and hence oxygen delivery is one of the primary goals in the management of the critically ill surgical patient. The main predeterminant of oxygen delivery is cardiac output; therefore, monitoring and therapeutic manipulation of cardiac output are essential components of critical care practice. Cardiac output is, in turn, determined by preload, cardiac function and compliance, and afterload (Fig. 8.1), all of which can be altered and monitored.

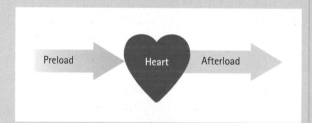

Figure 8.1 The determinants of cardiac output.

In most patients, clinical assessment, vital signs, urine output and simple tests such as core/ peripheral temperature gradients can provide a suitable evaluation of cardiovascular function. These will provide information on how well the cardiovascular system is fulfilling its basic function. The efficacy of the system in delivering oxygen and nutrients to the tissues, and removing carbon dioxide and other products of tissue metabolism, depends upon the production of a cardiac output sufficient to meet the demands of tissue metabolism. Clearly, this is highly variable depending on how well (or ill) a patient is. Furthermore, the cardiac output must be regionally matched to the metabolic needs of individual organs.

In critically ill patients, deviation from the normal ranges of any of these components of cardiac output can occur unexpectedly, rapidly and with little to see clinically in the early stages of deterioration. Clinical assessment alone may well be inadequate and the accuracy of estimation of volume status compared to more intensive monitoring techniques may be as low as 30%. Objective measurements showing change should be detected as early as possible to allow rapid corrective therapy before vital organ damage has occurred. Modern monitoring equipment can provide rapid, accurate and reproducible measurements of cardiovascular performance and the effects of treatment.

Cardiovascular therapy in the critically ill aims to avoid tissue hypoxia and the degree to which one must go to monitor the adequacy of the cardiovascular system in achieving this goal varies with severity of illness and complexity of the case. Organs vary in their ability to maintain their own perfusion (through autoregulation);

generally, measurements relate the total body picture, rather than adequacy of perfusion of specific viscera. Certain organs, notably the gut, are prone to hypoxia and this hypoxia may continue to drive the inflammatory process (including multiple organ failure) even once the initial causal factors have been dealt with. To overcome this, one approach has been to try and ensure that the critically ill patient with multiple organ failure has a circulation that provides an oxygen delivery which is, if anything, greater than normal, thus minimising the chance of occult hypoxia. A related approach has been to monitor plasma lactate level and/or negative BE on the grounds that elevated values of these suggest that tissue hypoxia may be present. An alternative strategy is to try and measure specific visceral perfusion (such as that of the intestine) by techniques such as tonometry. There is much to be said for pursuing similar objectives, at an appropriate level, in all unwell patients and particularly in the pre-operative preparation of the critically ill surgical patient.

In broad terms, the indications for intensive monitoring of the cardiovascular system are:

- failure to restore promptly and maintain cardiovascular homeostasis with simple techniques (i.v. fluids, surgery, non-invasive blood pressure, pulse oximetry)
- during procedures which may give rise to rapid or profound changes in preload or afterload
- during treatment with vaso-active drugs which influence preload, afterload or myocardial function, to monitor response to treatment and guide management strategies
- in any patient who has, or is at risk of developing, a low perfusion state from any cause.

The parameters that can be monitored include:
- blood pressure
- CVP
- cardiac output or CI.

## MEASUREMENT OF BLOOD PRESSURE

Non-invasive intermittent measurements of arterial blood pressure can be performed using an automated sphygmomanometer. However, non-invasive readings can be erroneous if size or positioning of the cuff is incorrect. Automated devices are useful to demonstrate trends in blood pressure and are reliable in most stable patients. In more unstable patients, more accurate readings are required using invasive techniques, whereby mechanical energy of blood pressure changes are converted to electrical energy using a transducer, allowing continuous monitoring on a screen. CVP monitoring utilises the same principles and shares the same potential pitfalls as arterial pressure monitoring.

### TRANSDUCERS

While the physical principles of how these individual measurements are made are beyond the scope of this course, certain basic scientific principles apply. Changes in any parameter to be measured must be detected accurately with sufficient sensitivity, over the range required, at a suitable frequency response often from inaccessible sites and converted by a transducer so that the signals vary in proportion to the changes in the parameters under study. A transducer converts the mechanical energy of pressure changes to electrical energy in a manner such that the electrical output of the transducer varies directly with the change in pressure. An example of this kind of system is shown in Fig. 8.2.

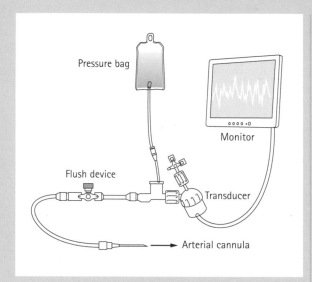

Figure 8.2 Signal transduction from an arterial cannula.

The pressure wave is transmitted from the artery (in this case) to the transducer through relatively rigid tubing. The transducer converts the mechanical signal to an electronic one, displayed on the monitor. The three-way tap on the transducer allows zeroing. Patency of the cannula is maintained by a slow constant flush of heparinised saline under pressure and most systems incorporate a button for bolus flushing to clear any debris and improve the signal.

The electrical signals must be displayed and processed so that derived results may be calculated. The measurement system must be zeroed and calibrated. If pressure is measured, this should be done with the transducer level relative to the point within the patient at which the pressure is to be measured. Care should be taken to minimise the interference and damping of the measurement signal to ensure optimal signal to noise ratio. Failure to zero or calibrate will produce erroneous results. This can also happen when the cannula or catheter is kinked, abuts the vessel wall or is partly occluded by clot.

## SAFEGUARDS

Before considering the individual techniques, one should be aware of certain ground rules common to all procedures used during invasive monitoring methods:

- a sound knowledge of relevant practical anatomy
- competency in the technique of insertion of the line
- the procedure should be explained to the patient
- all procedures must be performed using aseptic technique
- contra-indications and complications must be known
- the benefit accrued must exceed the risks of the procedure
- the patient must be in the care of people who know how to manage the lines, all of which must be Luer-locked to prevent disconnection
- all lines should be clearly labelled and injections into or sampling from lines ONLY performed at designated sites
- attendants should be familiar with the monitors to ensure that the data derived from them are accurate
- lines must be dressed aseptically and changed at appropriate intervals.

## ARTERIAL PRESSURE MONITORING

A peripheral artery can be cannulated either to allow continuous measurement of arterial blood pressure by connecting the cannula to a transducer, or to allow for repeated sampling of arterial blood for analysis. The radial artery is the most frequent anatomical site, followed by the dorsalis pedis artery, and a 20G or 22G sized cannula is used. The brachial and femoral arteries should be avoided if possible because of lack of collaterals and, in the case of the femoral site, the risk of sepsis.

When using the radial artery, always check for ulnar flow supply to the palmar arch using Allen's test prior to cannulation (Fig. 8.3). Local sepsis and coagulopathy are the main contra-indications while complications include haematoma, thrombosis, distal ischaemia, intimal damage, false aneurysm formation, disconnection and injection of irritant drugs. Samples from arterial cannulae should be taken aseptically and the line flushed and re-sealed afterwards. After cannulation of the artery, the cannula should be connected to a continuous-flush device containing heparinised saline under pressure which maintains patency and allows blood pressure changes to be conducted without letting blood flow out of the artery into the line.

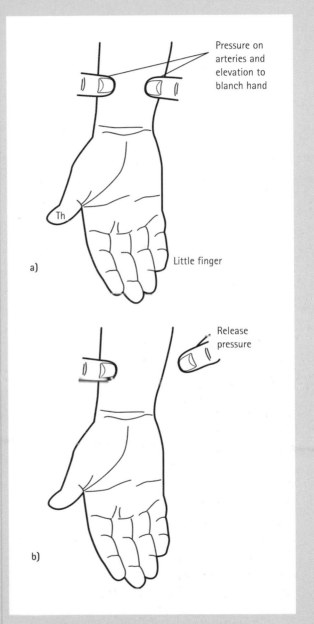

Figure 8.3 Allen's test. Blanch the hand by clenching the fist then simultaneously occlude radial and ulnar arteries at the wrist. An adequate pink flush of the hand on release of the ulnar pressure confirms an adequate ulnar supply to the palmar arterial arches.

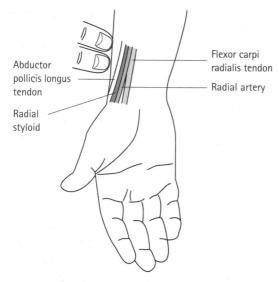

Abductor pollicis longus tendon

Radial styloid

Flexor carpi radialis tendon

Radial artery

## TECHNIQUE FOR RADIAL ARTERIAL PUNCTURE/CANNULATION

### Position and palpate
- position the hand and yourself comfortably, with adequate light and assistance
- palpate the artery with 2 fingers
- feel and imagine its course above and below the point of entry
- insert at 45°, avoiding the superficial vein which often overlies.

### Puncture
- advance needle tip in a linear fashion – do NOT wiggle it around!
- if you miss, re-palpate and search in a systematic fashion with further straight insertions
- let syringe fill and withdraw
- pressure haemostasis – 5 min.

### Cannulation: the Seldinger technique
- puncture as above
- advance guide wire
- railroad cannula
- check backflow and secure cannula
- connect transducer and flushing set-up.

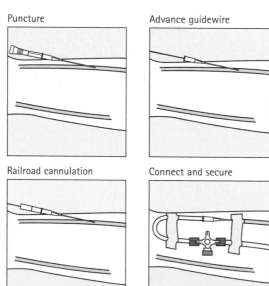

Puncture

Advance guidewire

Railroad cannulation

Connect and secure

Figure 8.4 Technique for radial arterial puncture/cannulation.

If the arterial cannula is to be used for pressure monitoring, it is connected via a relatively short length of rigid tubing to a 3 way tap, flush device and transducer. Check that the transducer is zeroed, calibrated at the correct level and that the lines contain no air bubbles, which would cause damping of the signal. The arterial waveform gives real-time information about the blood pressure and heart rate, but also modern computer algorithms can transform pressure changes into shifts in stroke volume or cardiac output. Often these need to be calibrated by an independent mechanism in order to compensate for the different levels of vascular compliance seen between and within patients. The morphology of the individual waveform can also give information with regards to the systemic vascular resistance and cardiac contractility in both normal and pathological conditions. In particular, a sharp peaked up-swing and down-swing with a low dicrotic notch can reflect significant hypovolaemia, but it is dangerous to draw such conclusions unless the system is adequately damped (Fig. 8.5).

The changes in the arterial pressure trace with the fluctuations in intrathoracic pressure during artificial mechanical ventilation can be used to determine patients who will respond to a fluid challenge by increasing their stroke volume. These changes can be characterised either by the systolic pressure variation, the pulse pressure variation or, nowadays when combined with a cardiac output monitor, the stroke volume variation.

## CENTRAL VENOUS PRESSURE MEASUREMENT

CVP measurement is one of the most commonly used monitoring tools in critical care, indicating preload of pulmonary circulation and a rough guide to systemic preload given a number of provisos. The CVP is simply the pressure within the SVC as it enters the right atrium, and reflects the ability of the right heart to accept and deliver circulating volume. The CVP is influenced by various factors, including venous return, right heart compliance, intrathoracic pressure and

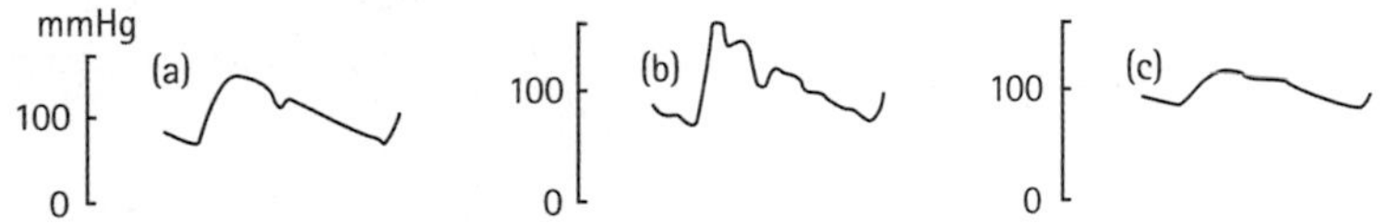

Figure 8.5 Arterial waveforms showing influence of damping:
a) adequately damped; b) underdamped; c) overdamped.

## CENTRAL VEIN CANNULATION

### Infraclavicular subclavian route

- tilt the patient 20° head down, arms by the side and head turned away from the side of entry
- make a skin nick and insert the cannula 1–2 cm below the mid point of the clavicle
- advance horizontally towards the suprasternal notch – remember, advance needle tip in a linearfashion – do NOT wiggle it around
- try and visualise the anatomy beneath as you do it – think where your needle tip is, particularly in relation to clavicle and pleura, and the narrow gap between clavicle and first rib, where the subclavian artery and vein run
- if you miss, search in a systematic fashion with further straight insertions, trying to picture where the vein is most likely to be
- when venous blood is aspirated freely, remove syringe and insert the guide wire

- leave enough guide wire outside to let you railroad the catheter over it without losing the wire inside the patient
- advance the catheter to a previously measured point, so the tip lies in the distal SVC
- secure the catheter and check its position by chest X-ray.

### Ultrasound image of the jugular vein and carotid artery

- using ultrasound, the vein is located at the medial border of sternomastoid, at the level of the thyroid cartilage and anterolateral to the carotid artery
- displace the artery medially and, under ultrasound guidance, advance the needle through a skin nick
- advance inferiorly at 30° to the skin, parallel to the artery but lateral: this is often towards the ipsilateral nipple
- puncture and proceed as above.

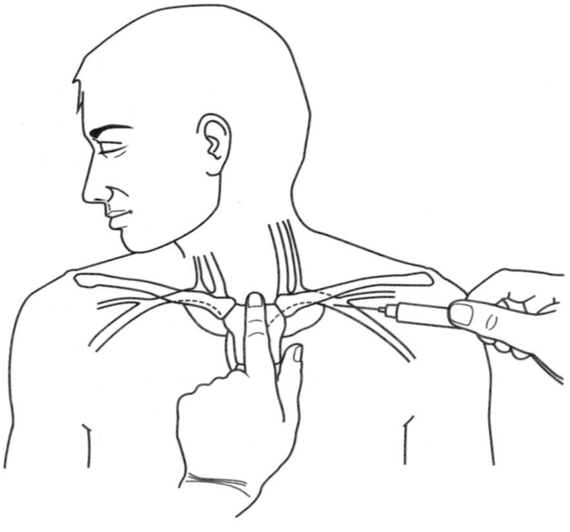

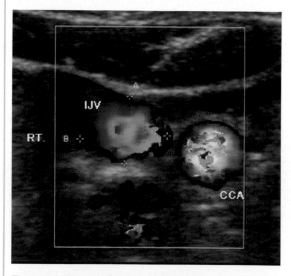

Figure 8.6a Infraclavicular subclavian vein cannulation using the Seldinger technique.

Figure 8.6b Ultrasound image of the jugular vein and carotid artery

patient position. While absolute measurements of CVP are useful (with the normal range 0–8 mmHg or 0–10 cmH$_2$O), often the trend in CVP, and response to fluid challenge or therapeutic manoeuvre is more important. This is particularly useful when trying to deduce the cause of shock (see Chapter 7).

## CVP ACCESS

The route for access to the central venous circulation depends on the skill and experience of the operator and the presence of site-specific contra-indications such as local sepsis, coagulopathy, abnormal anatomy, operative site and previous vein usage. While the techniques are illustrated in Figure 8.6a, it should be noted that the UK National Institute for Health and Clinical Excellence (NICE) recommends that ultrasound imaging should be used to guide placement of central venous catheters into the internal jugular vein in elective situations. NICE further recommends that all those involved in placing central venous catheters should undertake training to achieve competence in the use of ultrasound for this purpose. Ideally, ultrasound should also be used in emergency cases, though the anatomical landmark method is still recommended for the subclavian route.

The internal jugular site is advantageous in terms of a lower rate of complications, but is uncomfortable and difficult to dress. The subclavian route entails a higher risk, in particular the risk of pneumothorax and intrathoracic bleeding, which can be difficult to control.

## PRACTICE POINT

*No-one inexperienced in the technique of central venous catheterisation should undertake the procedure.*

## CVP MEASUREMENT

The best zero reference point, which represents the level of the SVC, is the mid-axillary line at the 4th intercostal space, with the patient supine. The alternative, the 2nd intercostal space at the sternal edge, represents a point about 5 cm above the atrium. For readings to be comparable at separate times, they should always be taken from the same point. The pressure may be measured using either a liquid manometer filled with sterile dextrose 5% or by an electronic transducer reading over a suitable pressure range in centimetres of water (Fig. 8.7).

The 'water' manometer is cheap, effective and simple and can be used on ordinary wards but does not respond to rapid changes in pressure. Its response time is, however, sufficiently fast to show the fluctuation in CVP with inspiration (fall in pressure) and expiration (rise in pressure), a change which confirms that the manometer is reflecting the normal change in CVP with fluctuation of intra-thoracic pressure. The electronic transducer is faster and the analysis of the signal produced allows the mean pressure to be displayed taking into account the variation with the respiratory cycle. The set up of the transducer is identical to that for arterial pressure measurement.

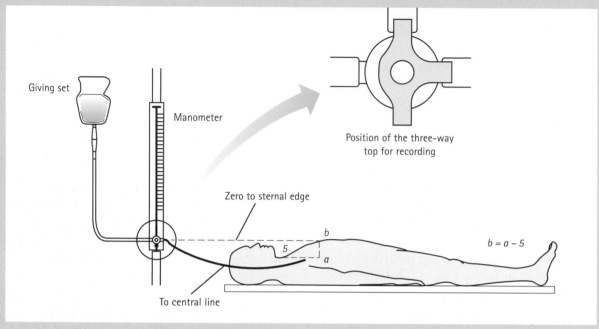

Figure 8.7 **Liquid manometer for CVP.**

## CVP WAVEFORM

The CVP waveform has a characteristic pattern that reflects changes in atrial pressure during the cardiac cycle as shown in Fig. 8.8.

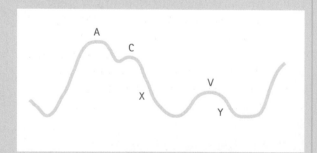

Figure 8.8 **The CVP waveform.** A wave, atrial contraction; C wave, bulging of the tricuspid valve into the right atrium; X descent, atrial relaxation; V wave; rise in atrial pressure prior to tricuspid valve opening; and Y descent, atrial emptying.

## INDICATIONS FOR CVP MEASUREMENT

- fluid replacement therapy for hypovolaemia when conventional access is not possible, when concern exists about over-transfusion or when there is uncertainty about fluid volume status. Central vein cannulation is NOT advocated as a primary route of access because of the risk of complications and low flow rates achievable (remember Poiseille's law)
- to measure the effect of vaso-active drugs on venous capacitance, particularly vasodilators
- to aid diagnosis of right ventricular failure, when a high pressure will be seen in the presence of poor cardiac output.

**PRACTICE POINT**

*CVP does not 'equal' intravascular volume and is not an indicator of left ventricular function.*

## PITFALLS IN PRACTICE

- inaccurate readings as a result of failure of zeroing or calibration, placement of the cannula tip in the right ventricle, tricuspid regurgitation and incompetence, A–V dissociation and nodal rhythms
- variations in intravascular volume, sympathetic tone, cardiac output, intrathoracic pressure (particularly during positive pressure ventilation) may lead to a false impression of a much higher right ventricular filling pressure than is actually present (Fig. 8.9)
- before using the line and acting on measurements made, always check for easy aspiration of blood, pressure fluctuation with respiration and confirmation of position on X-ray
- complications of central line insertion are numerous and relate to damage to the veins themselves and adjacent structures. Complications include rupture of vessel and haemorrhage with local haematoma or haemothorax, tension pneumothorax (particularly if the patient is on positive pressure ventilation), air embolism, extravascular catheter placement, knotting of catheters, catheter breakage, catheter misplacement, neurapraxia, arterial puncture, lymphatic puncture, tracheobronchial puncture and sepsis. Do not underestimate the potential severity of central line sepsis.

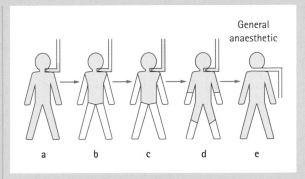

Figure 8.9 CVP and intravascular volume: pitfalls in the shocked surgical patient: a, normal; b, shocked but compensating (by peripheral vasoconstriction) with low CVP; c, rapid re-fill and (temporarily) high CVP; d, redistribution and falling CVP as degree of compensatory vasoconstriction lessens; and e, general anaesthesia with vasodilatation, loss of compensation and very low CVP

All staff involved in the care of patients with central venous access should be familiar with the 'saving lives high impact care bundle for central venous catheters'. The Health Act 2006 Code of Practice states that NHS organisations must audit key policies and procedures for infection prevention. The high-impact intervention approach to central venous catheters provides a focus on elements of the care process to prevent catheter-associated infections. These comprise aspects regarding line insertion, including aseptic techniques, skin preparation and hand hygiene, and on going care of the line, including regular inspection, aseptic techniques and regular replacement of administration sets.

## MEASUREMENTS OF CARDIAC OUTPUT/CARDIAC INDEX

In shock states, the delivery of oxygen to the tissues is at least as important as the level of systemic arterial pressure. Global oxygen delivery is a product of cardiac output and arterial oxygen content. Cardiac output is, therefore, a pivotal variable in the management of the critically ill surgical patient.

The understanding of the relationship between cardiac output and other parameters allows an estimate of systemic vascular resistance, using the following equation:

Cardiac output = Driving pressure (MAP–CVP)/systemic vascular resistance

Therefore, with a measurement of cardiac output, MAP and CVP, an estimate of SVR can be calculated and the combination of variables used to guide rational decisions about volume resuscitation and vasoactive therapies.

The pulmonary artery catheter (PAC or Swan–Ganz catheter) has long been the gold standard for advanced haemodynamic monitoring. Pulmonary artery pressure and pulmonary artery occlusion (or 'wedge') pressure can be used to monitor right heart function and preload of the systemic circulation. This is largely achieved using thermodilution techniques and a thermistor on the PAC. However, it is highly invasive with significant risks of serious complications and less invasive cardiac output monitors are becoming more available, translating into a declining use on the critical care unit. Cardiac indexing corrects any variable for patient size (Table 8.1).

### TABLE 8.1

#### VARIABLES DERIVED FROM CARDIAC OUTPUT MEASUREMENTS

**Systemic vascular resistance (SVR)**
- If too high (vasoconstriction), tissue hypoperfusion is likely
- If too low, maintenance of an adequate mean blood pressure will be difficult

**Stroke volume (SV), stroke index (SI)**
- A major determinant of cardiac output and governable by preload

**Left ventricular stroke work index (LVSWI)**
- An index of the function of the systemic side of the heart

**Oxygen delivery ($DO_2$)**
- An index of the oxygen delivered to all tissues

**Oxygen uptake ($VO_2$)**
- Index of oxygen consumption

### NON-INVASIVE MEASUREMENT OF CARDIAC FUNCTION

There are several less invasive techniques, including trans-oesophageal Doppler (TOD), echocardiography, pulse contour cardiac output with indicator dilution (PiCCO) and lithium indicator dilution calibration system (LiDCO™).

*Trans-oesophageal Doppler*
TOD uses the Doppler shift principle to make measurements of blood velocity in the descending aorta. A disposable Doppler probe contained at the tip of a 90 cm x 5.5 mm probe is passed down the oesophagus to lie at the level of the

descending aorta (around 35–45 cm) and rotated until the arterial waveform is displayed. This appears as a triangular shaped waveform since the shift signal is displayed as a velocity/time plot. The shape of the waveform provides information on preload, stoke volume and afterload (Fig 8.10). The area under the curve represents the stroke volume flowing through the descending aorta and applying a factor determined from the patient's age, height and weight allows the stroke volume to be calculated. A number termed the corrected flow time (FTc) is calculated: it is low in hypovolaemia and may be used to derive SVR. The disadvantage of the TOD is that the patient must be anaesthetised and intubated to tolerate the probe. It cannot be used in patients who have coarctation of the aorta or who are on intra-aortic balloon pumps.

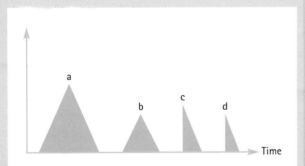

Figure 8.10 Stylised TOD waveforms for vascular abnormality: a, best waveform, normal configuration; b, failing left ventricle – decreased waveform height and low peak velocity. Giving inotropes increases waveform height and restores velocity; c, hypovolaemia – narrow waveform base with decreased FTc (giving volume lengthens flow time and widens waveform base); and d, high systemic vascular resistance/afterload – reduced waveform height and narrow base.

*Trans-thoracic and trans-oesophageal echocardiography*
Bedside echocardiography is becoming increasingly available as the hardware becomes more portable and more affordable. The main role in critical care is the assessment of preload and cardiac contractility before and after intervention, and the diagnosis of major cardiac structural abnormalities (pericardial tamponade, severe valvular and regional wall motion abnormalities).

*Indicator dilution and pulse contour analysis*
Instead of measuring temperature changes in the pulmonary artery, which requires a PAC, a thermistor can be placed in the systemic arterial circulation. PiCCO calculates cardiac output from a peripheral arterial cannula providing beat-to-beat information to a computer, which in turn follows the heart rate and pressure waveform and integrates the area under the curve. The accuracy of the method is improved as the cannula contains a sensitive thermistor allowing thermodilution. The small drop in the temperature of arterial blood that follows the injection of a bolus of ice-cold saline into a central vein is proportional to cardiac output. The thermodilution measurement is used to calibrate the continuous cardiac output monitoring software which calculates changes in cardiac output by analysing the pulse contour of the arterial waveform. PiCCO requires recalibration at regular intervals and becomes unreliable when the arterial waveform is suboptimal, for example with a kinked line, air or blood clots in the system or any other cause of a damped trace.

Other indicators can be used to replace thermodilution techniques. Lithium chloride, for example, is injected into a central vein and the lithium concentrations are subsequently analysed with an ion-sensitive electrode (LiDCO™).

Here, the blood can be sampled from a normal peripheral arterial line. Several drugs interfere with the lithium analysis and lithium is contra-indicated in some patients. As in thermodilution, lithium-dilution is combined with continuous pulse contour analysis and similar recalibration requirements and issues with damped arterial traces apply.

## CARDIOVASCULAR SUPPORT USING VASO–ACTIVE DRUGS

In the normal heart, cardiac output is determined by preload, afterload, heart rate, rhythm, contractility and balance of oxygen demand and supply. If the heart is damaged, for a given preload or afterload, cardiac output will decrease. This can be represented graphically either by pressure–volume loops or by the more familiar Frank Starling curve (see Chapter 7, Fig. 7.2).

## TABLE 8.2

### ACTION OF INOTROPIC AGENTS

| | Receptor | Effect | Clinical use |
|---|---|---|---|
| Noradrenaline | $\alpha$-adrenoceptor agonist | Arteriolar vasoconstriction | Septic shock with low SVR |
| Adrenaline | $\alpha$- and ß-adrenoreceptor agonist, predominantly ß1-adrenoreceptor at low dose | Positive inotropic and chronotropic. Vascoconstricts at high doses | Wide-spread in conditions of low cardiac output |
| Dopamine | $\alpha$- and ß-adrenoreceptors. Dopamine (DA) 1 and 2 receptors | Low dose: splanchnic vasodilation, increased renal and hepatic blood flow (DA1). High dose: vasoconstriction | Used as first choice inotrope in some HDUs |
| Dopexamine | DA1, DA2 and ß-adrenoreceptor agonist | Increases splanchnic blood flow | Controversial – in peri-operative optimisation |
| Dobutamine | Similar to dopamine | Reduces SVR and increases cardiac output | Cardiogenic shock |

Invasive cardiovascular monitoring collects the data which allows the construction of such curves so that the effects of varying preload, afterload, inotropes, etc. can be accurately recorded, ensuring that therapy is producing an objective improvement in the patient's cardiovascular status. The curves are time consuming to plot and often variations in fluid loading, vasodilatation and inotropic support are taken on the basis of repeated or continuous CI measurements.

If the CI remains low after correcting any hypovolaemia with a fluid challenge, inotropic or other vaso-active drugs are used with the aim of optimising myocardial contractility by balancing myocardial oxygen supply and demand. Accurate measurements of derived variables can predict probable therapeutic regimens.

Drugs that increase cardiac output and ejection fraction are known as inotropes. Ideally, in addition to these properties, they should reduce afterload and preload, resulting in decreased trans-ventricular wall tension, promoting coronary blood flow, increasing myocardial oxygen delivery and reducing oxygen consumption. Regrettably, the ideal inotrope does not exist but the most commonly used are adrenaline, noradrenaline and dobutamine. They all act by providing an upward left shift in the Starling curve as shown in Figure 7.2. Noradrenaline has a specific use in septic shock as a vasopressor: it is used to increase and maintain SVR within the normal range.

Vasodilators such as sodium nitroprusside or nitrates are of use when pulmonary oedema occurs in heart failure, although they can produce a reflex tachycardia if the blood pressure falls. Occasionally, both inotropes and vasodilators are used in combination (*e.g.* adrenaline and nitroglycerine in severe LVF).

Inotropes and vasodilators can only be used safely where a full range of monitoring is available. They should never be used on ordinary surgical wards and NEVER in the presence of hypovolaemia. Their dose ranges, modes of delivery, etc. are outside the scope of this course; your task is to recognise the clinical conditions that mandate their use and refer the patient to the appropriate level of care.

## SUMMARY
- adequate cardiovascular function is a pre-requisite for survival
- to determine cardiovascular function accurately and to control manipulative therapy, invasive monitoring is necessary
- all techniques have complications
- the monitoring utilised should be appropriate to the specific case in question.

# 9

# Renal failure, prevention and management

This chapter will help you to:

- understand the functions of the kidney
- anticipate and predict patients at risk of developing acute renal failure
- outline the initial management of a patient with acute renal failure and associated life-threatening emergencies
- know the common causes of acute kidney injury in the critically ill surgical patient and the five rules of renal failure
- be aware of the implications of chronic kidney disease in the surgical patient.

Abnormal renal function is common in surgical patients and poor urine output is one of the most common reasons for a trainee being called to see a patient. The kidneys have a wide range of functions and play a vital role in homeostasis. In the context of the critically ill patient, they can also be seen as 'bilateral retroperitoneal indicators of cardiovascular stability'.

Acute renal failure (ARF) in critically ill patients is associated with a mortality of around 20% and is often preventable, particularly with attention to careful fluid balance. It is the responsibility of the surgical team to anticipate and prevent ARF where possible. When it occurs, treatment is essentially supportive but the team must be vigilant for the life-threatening complications (hyperkalaemia, pulmonary oedema) and know how and when to refer for renal replacement therapy.

## FUNCTIONS OF THE KIDNEY

The primary functions of the kidney are:
- elimination of water-soluble waste products of metabolism other than carbon dioxide
- elimination of water-soluble drugs
- fluid and electrolyte homeostasis
- acid–base balance
- blood pressure control: renin–angiotensin system
- endocrine function: erythropoietin and vitamin D production

## PHYSIOLOGY OF RENAL FUNCTION

The kidney regulates fluid and electrolytes by filtration, secretion and re-absorption. Renal blood flow is around 20% of cardiac output (1000 ml/min in an adult) and renal plasma flow (RPF) is approximately 600 ml/min. The glomerulus filters 125 ml/min of renal plasma. This glomerular filtration rate (GFR) is a much more reliable marker of renal function than plasma creatinine. Most of this fluid is re-absorbed, with only 1% passed as urine (0.5–1 ml/kg/h). The kidney autoregulates its plasma flow over a wide range of mean arterial pressure (MAP). However at low MAP, RPF and GFR become supply dependent and urine output decreases – this is the kidney protecting itself from further reduction in perfusion pressure (Fig. 9.1). This is reversible in the short term but the kidney is much more vulnerable to other insults, particularly the tubular cells deep in the medulla, which is more poorly perfused than the cortex.

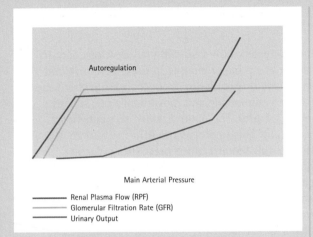

Figure 9.1 **Autoregulation maintains a steady glomerular filtration rate through a wide range of renal perfusion pressures.**

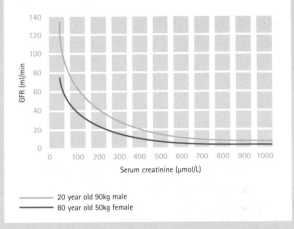

Figure 9.2 **The glomerular filtration rate steadily decreases with age, but this is not evident in raised creatinine until a relatively low level is reached.**

The plasma creatinine level and GFR are inversely related. If the plasma creatinine level drifts outside the normal range, the GFR may already be 50% of normal. It is important to recognise that a borderline creatinine may pose an increased risk of ARF, particularly in the elderly as the GFR decreases with age (Fig. 9.2).

## PRACTICE POINT

- *normal adult urine output is 1 ml/kg/h*
- *oliguria is < 400 ml/day (< 17 ml/h)*
- *anuria is < 100 ml/day.*

## RENAL FAILURE

There are 5 golden rules of renal failure in the surgical patient:

1. *The kidneys cannot function without adequate perfusion.*
2. *Renal perfusion is dependent on adequate blood pressure.*
3. *A surgical patient with poor urine output usually requires more fluid.*
4. *Absolute anuria is usually due to urinary tract obstruction.*
5. *Poor urine output in a surgical patient is not a frusemide deficiency.*

## CASE SCENARIO 9.1

8 hours following an elective abdominal aortic aneurysm repair, a 68-year-old man develops oliguria despite receiving 100 ml of 0.9% saline per hour and with no major change in pulse rate or blood pressure. There have been no obvious signs of haemorrhage or excess loss from the nasogastric tube. The CVP is 10 cmH$_2$O but the HDU nurse feels the trace is unreliable and 'positional', and suggests the patient is sub-optimally perfused. Haemoglobin is 11.1 g/dl. The junior trainee recommends a dose of frusemide (80 mg i.v.) to improve the urine output. This improves the urine output to 100 ml for 2 h, after which it falls again to 20 ml/h. The on-call senior trainee prescribes a further dose of frusemide (40 mg i.v.) by telephone. This has no effect and the ICU consultant is contacted. He re-sites the CVP line and the measurement is found to be very low. Immediate circulatory volume expansion, however, does not restore urinary output. By the next day, the plasma creatinine and urea levels have risen rapidly and renal replacement therapy is required. The patient has a long and complicated course and dies of multiple organ failure 3 weeks later.

### LEARNING POINTS

- adequate renal perfusion is the critical factor – this is often simply achieved with careful attention to fluid balance
- insensible and tissue fluid losses continue after surgery – postoperative hypovolaemia is common and may not be caused by acute postoperative haemorrhage
- CVP readings complement clinical assessment and are not a substitute
- consider advice from nursing staff
- frusemide will not salvage renal function in a hypovolaemic patient – the window of opportunity for successful simple treatment is narrow
- the five rules of renal failure would have helped in the management of this patient.

# ACUTE RENAL FAILURE

## DEFINITION

Acute renal failure is a biochemical diagnosis defined as an acute increase in serum creatinine resulting from injury or an inability to excrete the nitrogenous and other waste products of metabolism.

There are over 20 different classifications of acute renal failure – the Acute Kidney Injury (AKI) classification is the system currently in vogue. AKI is recognised as one of three clinical scenarios:

1. *An abrupt (within 48 h) reduction in kidney function defined as an absolute increase in serum creatinine level of $\geq 26.4$ mmol/l (0.3 mg/dl), or*

2. *A percentage increase in serum creatinine level of $\geq 50\%$ (1.5-fold from baseline), or*

3. *A reduction in urine output (documented oliguria of < 0.5 ml/kg/h for > 6 h).*

These criteria should be applied in the context of the clinical presentation and following adequate fluid resuscitation and exclusion of obstruction.

There are three stages of AKI based on GFR and urine output, detailed in Table 9.1.

## EPIDEMIOLOGY

The incidence of ARF very much depends on the population being studied, from 5% of general acute hospital admissions, to 10% of unplanned surgical admissions to ICU and 50% of those with septic shock.

## AETIOLOGY

There are a diverse number of causes of ARF, most usefully classified as pre-renal, intrinsic renal and post-renal (Table 9.2). In surgical patients, pre-renal failure is the most common aetiology (75%), followed by intrinsic renal and post-renal (20% and 5%, respectively).

### TABLE 9.1

THE STAGES OF THE ACUTE KIDNEY INJURY CLASSIFICATION

| Stage | GFR criteria | Urine output criteria |
|-------|--------------|----------------------|
| 1 | Increase in creatinine > 26.4 $\mu$mol/l or 1.5–2.0-fold from baseline | < 0.5 ml/kg/h over 6 h |
| 2 | Increase in creatinine 2–3-fold from baseline | < 0.5ml/kg/h over 12 h |
| 3 | Increase in creatinine 3-fold from baseline or serum creatinine > 354 mmol/l | < 0.3ml/kg/h over 24 h |

## TABLE 9.2

### COMMON CAUSES OF ACUTE RENAL FAILURE

**Pre-renal**
- Hypovolaemia
- Sepsis
- Low cardiac output

**Intrinsic renal**
- Acute tubular necrosis
- Ischaemic injury – hypoxia, hypoperfusion
- Nephrotoxic injury – endotoxins, drugs, contrast, pigments
- Abdominal compartment syndrome
- Hepatorenal syndrome

**Post-renal**
- Bladder outflow obstruction
- Bilateral ureteric obstruction

In pre-renal failure, the kidney is structurally and functionally intact but has reduced blood flow, hence GFR. Essentially, this is a reversible state if acted upon urgently but may progress to acute tubular necrosis (ATN) in hours. Intrinsic renal failure involves parenchymal damage. The renal vasculature, glomerular and tubulo-interstitium may all be affected. ATN is by far the commonest cause, which results from a combination of ischaemic and nephrotoxic injury. Post-renal failure results from obstruction and back pressure which disturbs tubular function. Relief of obstruction enables urine to flow but tubular function may be disturbed during the recovery period.

## MANAGEMENT OF RENAL FAILURE

In surgical patients, there are four common scenarios regarding renal failure:
- an elective patient at risk of renal failure (with or without pre-operative chronic renal impairment)
- acute renal impairment in a critically ill patient
- a patient with established renal failure
- a patient with chronic renal failure (CRF).

### PRE-OPERATIVE MANAGEMENT AND PREVENTION OF RENAL FAILURE

*Predict and protect*

It is essential to identify those at risk of developing peri-operative renal dysfunction, particularly those with pre-existing renal impairment. Common causes of CRF include: hypertension, diabetes, renal artery stenosis, glomerulonephritis and use of drugs (e.g. diuretics, ACE inhibitors, NSAIDs, aminoglycosides).

For elective procedures, it is sometimes prudent to delay surgery, investigate the cause of pre-existing renal impairment and look at measures to protect renal function, including a review of drug therapy and avoiding nephrotoxins such as contrast medium. Relevant investigations may include urinalysis, renal ultrasound and more detailed tests of split renal function such as a MAG3 scan. It is often worth seeking the opinion of a renal physician at an early stage. Ensure optimum peri-operative fluid balance and optimise the cardiovascular status – especially in terms of volume, avoiding hypotension and hypovolaemia. Diabetes should be closely controlled.

In the emergency setting, strict attention to fluid balance and maintenance of optimum cardiac output is essential with further avoidance of renal insults including nephrotoxic drugs and aggressive management of any sepsis. It is often a combination of factors that tip a patient into renal failure, in particular the combination of hypovolaemia, nephrotoxic drugs and sepsis, rather than one specific insult. In both the elective and emergency setting, those at risk should be reviewed regularly.

## MANAGEMENT OF ACUTE RENAL IMPAIRMENT

The principles of management revolve around the systematic CCrISP assessment protocol, with particular attention to:
- recognition and correction of respiratory and circulatory problems

## CASE SCENARIO 9.2

A 45-year-old previously healthy woman presents with jaundice and cholangitis. She has a pyrexia (38.4°C) and a tachycardia (115 bpm) but is normotensive. She is treated with intravenous antibiotics and fluids and her condition improves; an urgent ultrasound scan suggests stones in the common bile duct. An ERCP is booked for later in the week.

The ERCP proves difficult and adequate drainage of the common bile duct is not achieved. A PTC is scheduled for the following day but, 12 h after the ERCP, the patient becomes hypotensive and pyrexial. The serum amylase and an abdominal radiograph are normal. Treatment is started with oxygen, intravenous fluid challenges and the intravenous antibiotics are continued. She is transferred to the HDU and a CVP line inserted (+10 cmH$_2$O). The blood pressure is restored but the urine output remains poor and by the following morning the urea is 25.7 and creatinine 229. The patient is not on any nephrotoxic drugs.

It is clear that definitive treatment in the form of biliary drainage is needed urgently. An emergency PTC is arranged for later the same day. The PTC is performed by a consultant radiologist with an anaesthetist and an HDU nurse in attendance and with portable monitoring in place. Successful biliary drainage is achieved but the patient requires several days of haemofiltration on the HDU. She eventually makes a slow, but full, recovery, has a successful ERCP and subsequent elective laparoscopic cholecystectomy.

### LEARNING POINTS
- Multiple factors often contribute to acute renal failure in surgical critical care — biliary obstruction, sepsis and hypovolaemia are a potent combination.
- Patients with obstructive jaundice tend to be dehydrated and need adequate fluid therapy and clinical monitoring.
- Procedures such as ERCP and PTC can exacerbate hypovolaemia or sepsis in a number of ways and adequate peri-procedural antibiotics and intravenous fluids are needed in such cases — they are easily overlooked.
- Timely, definitive treatment of the underlying cause is usually the key to success.

- immediate identification and management of any life-threatening consequences of renal impairment
- exclusion of urinary tract obstruction if anuric
- careful search for, and correction of, the underlying cause
- help early from appropriate specialists.

## PRACTICE POINT

*Complete anuria means lower urinary tract/catheter obstruction until proven otherwise.*

## PATIENT ASSESSMENT

An accurate history is essential, supplemented by any information available from relatives, the patient's GP and the case notes. A note should be made of any factors that predispose the patient to increased risk of renal failure.

Frequently, there are no specific symptoms associated directly with ARF. Uraemic symptoms, commonly seen in chronic renal failure (such as anorexia, nausea, vomiting and itching) are rare. Signs may relate to the uraemic state particularly related to fluid overload and pulmonary oedema, but this may be attributed to other clinical problems especially in the multi-organ failure patient. A thorough, systematic examination is essential to identify any subtle signs of underlying disease, such as skin lesions in vasculitis, enlarged prostate and/or bladder and polycystic kidneys. A thorough and repeated assessment of intravascular volume should be performed. This can be difficult in the critically ill patient,

who may have adequate or excessive fluid but in the wrong compartment. The signs of hypovolaemia should be revised but remember that hypovolaemia can exist in the presence of normotension and significant extravascular oedema. Fluid overload may lead to an elevated blood pressure but, in particular, a raised JVP/CVP. Extravascular fluid overload may manifest as peripheral and pulmonary oedema, ascites and effusions.

## INVESTIGATIONS IN ARF

Dipstick urinalysis is mandatory in renal dysfunction. Marked proteinuria or microscopic haematuria with casts suggest a primary renal insult. Urine biochemistry and microbiology should also be considered, with biochemistry sometimes helping to distinguish between pre-renal and intrinsic renal failure (see below).

A renal ultrasound scan is also mandatory in any patient with ARF. This should be performed immediately in an anuric patient, if an obvious urinary tract obstruction is not detected clinically. Ultrasound will also provide information regarding renal size and blood flow.

Plain abdominal X-ray is rarely useful, but plain chest X-ray can reveal pulmonary oedema. Further radiological investigation should only be ordered after discussion with seniors, as it will often entail a contrast load and further renal insult. CT is the most useful investigation along with radionucleotide studies in terms of identifying problems with renal blood flow, renal function and obstruction.

A number of blood tests should be considered to complement routine biochemistry depending on the clinical scenario (Table 9.3).

## TABLE 9.3

### BLOOD TESTS TO COMPLEMENT ROUTINE BIOCHEMICAL ANALYSIS

FBC: to detect anaemia, infection

Routine biochemistry: urea, creatinine; check potassium

LFT: to recognise hepatorenal syndrome

Calcium phosphate: if associated malignancy, rhabdomyolysis or tumour lysis suspected

Creatine kinase: to detect rhabdomyolysis

C-reactive protein: as a measure of infection and/or inflammation

ABG and lactate: to assess hypoxia, acidosis and tissue/organ ischaemia

## TREATMENT

Look for a reversible cause and act urgently to:
- restore and maintain renal perfusion
- relieve any obstruction
- oxygenate the tubules
- remove/avoid toxins
- identify and treat any underlying cause.

## CHECKLIST

*Is it pre-renal failure?*
Consider the clinical scenario. Surgical patients often become hypovolaemic, for a variety of reasons. Often, oliguria can be corrected by restoring volume.

*Distinguish pre-renal from intrinsic renal failure due to ATN*
Classically, in pre-renal failure, the concentrating ability of the tubular system is retained producing urine with high osmolarity, high urea and creatinine and low sodium concentration. In ATN, a low osmolar urine with high sodium and low urea/creatinine is produced (Table 9.4 overleaf). Note there are many confounding variables and, in clinical practice, the full biochemical analysis is rarely performed.

*Restore renal perfusion with volume*
Aim to restore euvolaemia using 0.9% NaCl initially, and ensure regular monitoring of cardio-vascular parameters, particularly urine output. Once euvolaemic, give maintenance fluid to match urine output plus 30 ml and on going loss per hour. If there is no rapid response to restoration of circulating volume, central venous monitoring is required, probably with invasive circulatory monitoring and inotropic support.

There is no evidence to support the use of diuretics or dopamine in the prevention or treatment of renal impairment.

*Exclude post-renal obstruction*
Exclude post-renal obstruction with ultrasonography and treat accordingly.

*Distinguish between acute and chronic renal problems*
Ultrasound may reveal small kidneys (< 9 cm) with echo-bright parenchyma, suggesting chronic damage. The acutely injured, but normal, kidney will be echo bright due to oedema, but normal size and is more likely to recover. Acute or chronic renal failure is much less likely to recover.

## TABLE 9.4

### URINE VALUES IN PRE-RENAL AND INTRINSIC RENAL FAILURE

| Investigation | Pre-renal | Intrinsic renal |
| --- | --- | --- |
| Urinary specific gravity | > 1.020 | < 1.010 |
| Urinary sodium (mmol/l) | 10–20 | > 20 |
| Urinary osmolality (mosmol/l) | > 500 | < 350 |
| Urine/plasma osmolality ratio | > 2 | < 1.1 |
| Urine/plasma urea ratio | > 20 | < 10 |
| Urine/plasma creatinine ratio | > 40 | < 20 |
| Fractional sodium excretion | < 1% | > 1% |
| Renal failure index | < 1 | > 1 |

Note that: fractional sodium excretion = (urine/plasma sodium ratio)/(urine/plasma creatinine ratio) x 100, and renal failure index = (urine sodium)/(urine/plasma creatinine ratio).

*Oxygenate the tubules*
Give oxygen and maintain a saturation of greater than 95%. Also ensure that the Hb is greater than 7 g/dl.

*Exclude toxins*
Review the drug chart and avoid nephrotoxins including contrast medium. Common examples are aminoglycosides, NSAIDs, ACE inhibitors, opioids and ß-blockers. Any drug excreted by the kidney must have its dose altered when renal function is impaired to prevent toxic side effects. If in doubt, ask a pharmacist. Remember to test for pigments such as myoglobinuria and haemoglobinuria where appropriate.

Rhabdomyolysis is the breakdown of damaged muscle with release of myoglobin into the circulation. This commonly occurs following crush injuries and following acute limb ischaemia. Myoglobinuria is recognised as dark brown urine, which tests positive for myoglobin on urinalysis. Treatment includes aggressive volume expansion and sodium bicarbonate to alkalanise the urine, creating a diuresis and limiting the deleterious effect of acid breakdown products of myoglobin on renal tubules. This is only successful if recognised early and treated immediately.

## MANAGEMENT OF ESTABLISHED ARF

### INDICATIONS FOR DIALYSIS

If acute renal insufficiency fails to respond to the above measures and progresses to acute renal failure, renal replacement therapy (RRT) will be required. The indications for RRT are summarised in Table 9.5.

## TABLE 9.5

### INDICATIONS FOR RENAL REPLACEMENT THERAPY

**Absolute**
- Refractory hyperkalaemia (> 6 mmol/l)
- Refractory pulmonary oedema and fluid overload
- Uraemic encephalopathy

**Relative**
- Acidosis (pH < 7.2)
- Uraemia
- Pericarditis
- Toxin removal

Note that the threshold for RRT in uraemia is controversial and relates to the rapidity of rise as well as the absolute level of urea. A rise above 35 mmol/l unresponsive to other therapies is usually an absolute indication. RRT can be performed by dialysis or haemofiltration, depending on the clinical circumstances.

## HAEMODIALYSIS

Haemodialysis is a process by which low molecular weight solute equilibrates between a blood compartment and a dialysate compartment separated by a semipermeable membrane. Solute waste moves across the membrane down a concentration gradient (Fig. 9.3a). The dialysate contains normal solute, including sodium, calcium, magnesium and chloride in the appropriate concentration to maintain normal blood concentrations. Dialysis can be intermittent or continuous. Intermittent dialysis creates rapid changes in plasma osmolality and volume, making continuous methods more favourable in critically ill patients.

## HAEMOFILTRATION

In haemofiltration, there is a continuous convection of molecules across a permeable membrane (Fig. 9.b). The fluid that is removed is replaced with a buffered physiological solution. This is more effective in removing large quantities of fluid, but not as effective as dialysis at clearing smaller molecules. As with dialysis, filtration is usually performed using a continuous veno-venous method (CVVH). This method provides the least risk of significant intravascular fluid shifts and haemodynamic instability.

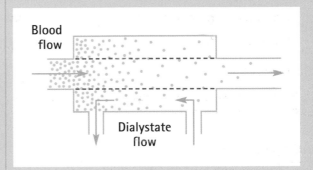

Figure 9.3a Dialysis

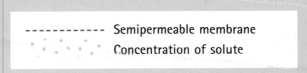

Semipermeable membrane

Concentration of solute

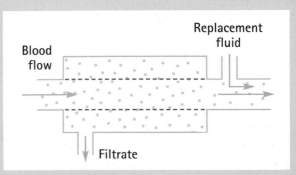

Figure 9.3b Haemofiltration

## MANAGEMENT OF LIFE-THREATENING COMPLICATIONS

### HYPERKALAEMIA

Acute hyperkalaemia ($K^+$ above 6.5 mmol/l) requires immediate treatment to prevent life-threatening cardiac dysrhythmia and VF/asystolic arrest. Rate of rise is also important: a rapid rise to 6 mmol/l is equally a cause for concern. There are usually no symptoms specific to a rise in potassium and clinical suspicion in the vulnerable patient is crucial.

Any underlying contributing cause should be identified and stopped, including blood transfusions, drugs that reduce renal potassium excretion (potassium sparing diuretics, ACE inhibitors, etc.), intravenous fluid containing potassium and potassium supplements.

An ECG should be performed. Hyperkalaemia may cause peaked T waves, absent P waves, widened QRS and ventricular arrhythmias. In the presence of ECG changes and a potassium above 6 mmol/l, emergency measures should be instituted to reduce $K^+$ levels temporarily, though this will only shift the potassium into the intracellular space. Immediate measures include (also see Table 9.6):

- commencing continuous cardiac monitoring
- insulin (10–20 units actrapid) in 100 ml 20% dextrose intravenously over 30 min
- sodium bicarbonate 50 mmol intravenously over 5–10 min
- 10% calcium gluconate intravenously (10–30 ml)
- Beta-2 agonist, *e.g.* nebulised or intravenous salbutamol.

**TABLE 9.6**

EMERGENCY THERAPY FOR HYPERKALAEMIA

| Drug | Mechanism of action | Pros and cons |
|---|---|---|
| Calcium gluconate (i.v. 10–30 ml of 10% solution) | Membrane stabilisation | Rapid effect but transient action |
| Insulin/dextrose (insulin [10–20 U actrapid] in 100 ml 20% dextrose i.v. over 30 min) | Drives potassium into cells | Rapid effect, intermediate action but needs central line |
| Sodium bicarbonate (50 mmol i.v. over 5–10 min followed by i.v. infusion of 1.26% or 1.4% solution at 100 ml/h) | Transfer of potassium into cells by exchange for hydrogen across membrane | Rapid effect – intermediate action, best with metabolic acidosis; beware sodium overload |
| Salbutamol (5–10 $\mu$g/min by intravenous infusion, or nebulised) | Transfer of potassium into cells | Rapid effect, short action; risk of tachycardia, vasodilator effect |

If, after emergency treatment, renal function is not improving, treatment should be introduced to reduce total body potassium. This can be achieved by: (i) dialysis (particularly if combined with fluid overload); or (ii) ion exchange resin (in the form of calcium resonium, 15 g 6–8-hourly or 30 g rectally; this binds potassium within the gut but is very unpleasant to take and is of limited benefit).

## PULMONARY OEDEMA

Pulmonary oedema presents as acute shortness of breath, associated with anxiety, tachycardia, tachypnoea, cool peripheries, and wide-spread crepitations/wheeze. If suspected, a chest X-ray should be performed immediately (if safe to do so). Sit the patient upright, stop all intravenous infusions, give high-flow oxygen and monitor saturations with a view to achieve $SaO_2$ of greater than 95%. Further treatment options include:

- intravenous diamorphine 2.5 mg for vasodilatory and anxiolytic effects
- intravenous GTN infusion, if systolic BP is greater than 100mmHg. Commence infusion at 2 mg/h and titrate upwards every 15 min
- intravenous frusemide, 250 mg in 50 ml saline over 1 h
- review regularly
- discuss higher level of support, particularly in the presence of: oligo/anuria, continued tachypnoea (> 30/min), signs of fatigue, respiratory failure ($PaO_2$ < 8 kPa, $PaCO_2$ > 7 kPa), acidosis (pH < 7.2).

## CHECKLIST WHEN MAKING A NEPHROLOGY REFERRAL

Expect to answer the following:
- clinical scenario – what do you think is going on?
- what is the pre-morbid state?
- what are the most recent creatinine, serum potassium and ABG results?
- what is the volume and cardiovascular status?
- what volumes of urine are they passing?
- what was the 'pre-insult' renal function?
- what does the ultrasonography show?
- what drugs are they on (in particular have they received any nephrotoxins)?

## PROGNOSIS AND RECOVERY

As individual nephrons recover, the kidney behaves as in chronic renal failure. Because only a proportion of the nephron mass has recovered, each nephron has a much higher solute load to excrete. There is, therefore, a major limitation in the kidneys' ability to conserve sodium, potassium, bicarbonate and water. With modern management of renal failure, it is unusual to see major problems with large fluid and electrolyte losses. The major exception is in postobstructive diuresis where losses need to be measured and replaced as appropriate. It is important that the recovering kidney is not exposed to further hypotensive or nephrotoxic insults. By 6 months, the kidney will normally have recovered to 85–90% of pre-morbid function, though some patients will invariably progress to CRF requiring permanent RRT or transplantation (10%).

Prognosis is often determined by the severity of the underlying incident that caused the ARF. However, in-hospital ARF due to ATN carries 20–30% mortality, most commonly due to infection or cardiovascular complications.

## CASE SCENARIO 9.3

You are asked to see a 75-year-old hypertensive diabetic woman on the ward who had a reversal of Hartmann's procedure 2 days ago. Her observations reveal a BP of 110/70, pulse 100 bpm, temperature 37.8°C, $O_2$ sats 89% (on air) and urine output of 20 ml for the past 3 hours. Her blood tests this morning are available: Hb 10.1, Ur 8, Cr 123, Na 130, K 5.0.

### WHAT ARE YOUR PRIORITIES AND WHAT OTHER INFORMATION DO YOU WANT TO KNOW?

* Follow the CCrISP protocol, in particular with regard to the renal dysfunction. This lady is unstable and needs careful monitoring. She may be developing acute renal failure.
* To restore renal perfusion, you should prescribe a fluid challenge (0.9% saline 1 l over 2 h) but you do not want her to develop pulmonary oedema.
* Oxygenate the tubules by sitting the patient up, give high flow oxygen and institute continuous $O_2$ monitoring.
* Review drugs for nephrotoxins. You stop an ACE inhibitor and NSAID.
* Regular observations (every 30 min) aiming for systolic BP of 130–140, BP < 100 bpm, $SaO_2$ > 95%, RR 12–15, and urine output of 30 ml/h. Set a time for review in 1–2 h.
* You would want to know the pre-operative blood pressure and serum creatinine, weight of the patient, plus fluid balance since surgery.

After the fluid challenge, you find the blood pressure has improved with a systolic pressure of 140, which is good for renal perfusion, although urine output is still poor at 20 ml in 2 h. The $SaO_2$ is 94% on supplemental oxygen and, worryingly, the respiratory rate has risen to 24/min.

### HOW WOULD YOU MANAGE THIS SITUATION NOW?

The findings suggest pulmonary oedema may be developing. Stop further fluid challenges. Perform a fluid assessment to look for evidence of fluid overload. You arrange a chest X-ray and ABGs, re-check U+Es.

The chest X-ray shows interstitial oedema, and ABG reveals an acidosis (pH 7.25, $PaO_2$ 9 kPa, $PaCO_2$ 4.5, BE-5, lactate 2) and the biochemistry is worse (Ur 12, Cr 148, Na 129, K 5.9).

### WHAT IS YOUR ASSESSMENT? WHAT SHOULD YOU DO?

It looks like she is now developing pulmonary oedema (interstitial oedema, hypoxaemia) and acute renal failure (Cr and K rising, metabolic acidosis). She needs a higher level of care than the ward. Discuss with HDU her organ failure and need for renal and respiratory support.

### LEARNING POINTS

* Predict and prevent renal failure by identifying the surgical patient at risk.
* Immediate management of renal failure requires close attention to fluid balance while recognising the risk of developing pulmonary oedema.
* Pulmonary oedema can be life-threatening and often requires a higher level of care with respiratory and renal support.

> **PRACTICE POINT**
>
> *Acute renal failure is not a cause of death unless a decision has been made not to treat the resultant uraemia. The cause of death is the underlying condition.*

## FUTURE DEVELOPMENTS

Creatinine and urine output are relatively insensitive markers of renal function and hence new 'biomarkers' are being sought to identify and predict those at risk of impending ARF, including neutrophil gelatinase-associated lipocalin, and kidney injury marker-1.

## CHRONIC RENAL FAILURE

CRF is defined as chronic irreversible loss of nephron mass resulting in permanent impairment of solute waste excretion. These patients are not necessarily requiring permanent RRT. By estimating the GFR using the Cockcroft Gault formula, 5% of the adult population will have sub-clinical stage 3 CRF (a GFR 30–60 ml/min). However, such patients deserve special attention to detail due to:

- significant risk of developing ARF
- multiple medications, especially cardiovascular drugs
- concomitant silent cardiovascular disease
- abnormal cardiovascular physiology – autonomic dysfunction reduces normal response to volume changes, especially diabetics
- abnormal gastrointestinal function – delayed transit, impaired absorption
- abnormal drug handling – impaired excretion requires dose modification; consult with pharmacy.

Patients who have CRF, therefore, have much less ability to compensate for circulatory stress and the effects of nephrotoxins. A simple example is the patient with significant CRF (creatinine of 300 mmol/l) who is fasted overnight prior to surgery. This will cause mild intravascular volume depletion. As there are far fewer nephrons, each has to carry increased solute and this acts as an osmotic diuretic that prevents concentration of the urine. This prevents maximum sodium and water retention until there has been a significant fall in glomerular filtration rate secondary to a contracted circulating volume. Thus, the patient becomes dehydrated and renal function diminishes further. Depriving patients with CRF of oral fluid for any significant length of time (greater than 4–6 h) should be avoided unless fluid is given intravenously.

Many patients with severe CRF will be chronically anaemic. Rapid transfusion will acutely impair renal function by altering the flow characteristics of the blood and is seldom necessary.

Patients with renal transplants must be managed in conjunction with their nephrologist or transplant centre. Skilled assistance will be required to manage their immunosuppression and reduce the likelihood of an acute rejection episode.

## SUMMARY

Predict and prevent renal failure, and remember the five rules of renal dysfunction in surgical patients:

- The kidneys cannot function without adequate perfusion.
- Renal perfusion is dependent on adequate blood pressure.
- A surgical patient with poor urine output usually requires more fluid.
- Absolute anuria is usually due to urinary tract obstruction.
- Poor urine output in a surgical patient is not a frusemide deficiency.

## FURTHER READING

### Acute Renal Failure

Hilton R. Acute renal failure. *BMJ* 2006; 333: 786–90.

Mehta RL, Kellum JA, Shah SV *et al.* Acute Kidney Injury Network: report of an initiative to improve outcomes in acute kidney injury. *Crit Care* 2007; 11: R31.

### Fluid assessment/management

Powell-Tuck J, Gosling P, Lobo DN *et al.* *British Consenus Guidelines on Intravenous Fluid Therapy for Adult Surgical Patients (GIFTASUP).* London: NHS National Library of Health, 2008.

*Oxford Handbook of Nephrology and Hypertension.* Oxford University Press, 2006.

# 10

## Peri-operative management of the surgical site

## OBJECTIVES

This chapter will help you to:

- recognise the difficulties of assessing the surgical patient postoperatively, especially on the ICU
- understand how the CCrISP system can be utilised to assess and manage problems associated with the surgical site effectively
- be aware of the presentation of common and/or serious complications in surgical patients and develop an approach to both their prevention and treatment
- develop an approach to the management of the surgical sites in the form of wounds, drains and stomas.

## INTRODUCTION

Surgery is a significant physiological insult, especially when performed for a critical presentation. The time following the procedure requires a plan of resuscitation and recovery in successful cases, but there is always a risk that complications may arise, including infection, haemorrhage, ischaemia or incomplete resolution of the original presentation. The challenge is to be able to recognise any deterioration early and intervene before the advent of organ failure and subsequent ICU requirement with its inherent high mortality risk. While recognising a deterioration in the immediate management, the history of the presentation or the operation notes may give a better guide to a likely cause, or allow successful intervention if events are predicted. The anticipation of problems is a great skill to acquire (see Table 10.1), allowing earlier and targeted intervention

to decrease the chance of deterioration. Significant deterioration may require ICU admission for resuscitation and monitoring; if organ failure ensures, the operative mortality can be in excess of 50%.

Whether on the ward or in a higher dependency area it is often difficult to assess the surgical site, especially within the abdomen. However, it is the surgical team's responsibility to ensure that there is appropriate monitoring and a management plan. This includes all components of the surgical site, including wound management and plans for drains, stomas or fistulae.

## PRACTICE POINT

TASK: *reflect on your last major operation. Consider what the potential complications were, and how these may present. If the patient did experience complications, were there things that could have been done to prevent these?*

## POSTOPERATIVE ASSESSMENT OF THE SURGICAL SITE

The end of an operation is equivalent to the 'decide and plan' component of the CCrISP assessment system. The desired expectation would be for the patient to be stable and progressing safely within a structured management plan. That plan begins with the operation note where the indication for the procedure, especially if in a critical pre-operative condition, and the essential findings should be clearly documented. The operative procedure and any difficulties encountered should be described. An operative diagram is often helpful to describe the internal and external anatomy, as well as representing

**TABLE 10.1**

EXAMPLES OF ANTICIPATED POSTOPERATIVE COMPLICATIONS
ASSOCIATED WITH INITIAL PRESENTATION

| Surgical presentation | Potential postoperative complication |
|---|---|
| Infarcted bowel from intestinal ischaemia | Further ischaemia causing anastomotic breakdown, abscess/collection, fistula formation |
| Ruptured abdominal aortic aneurysm | Open repair: reactive or secondary haemorrhage/abdominal compartment syndrome/ lower limb ischaemia/postoperative ileus<br>Endovascular repair: stent thrombosis and limb ischaemia/abdominal compartment syndrome/ renal impairment |
| Diverticular abscess and systemic sepsis | Anastomotic leak and recurrent sepsis<br>Intra-peritoneal abscess<br>Any inotropic support will increase risk of anastomotic leak or end stoma infarction |
| Penetrating abdominal trauma | Increased risk of sepsis/need for laparostomy if regular re-look laparotomy required<br>Risk of abdominal compartment syndrome |
| Appendicitis | Wound infection and abscess formation<br>Intra-peritoneal pelvic collection |
| Any presentation with co-morbid risk factors: age, obesity, smoking and diabetes | Task: consider these co-morbidities and the complications which might occur related to these factors. Then refer to Chapter 16 for further information |

the position of drains and stomas. Clear postoperative instructions must be written especially with regard to the management of drains or stomas and when or how to start feeding (see Case Scenario 10.1).

Also, a description of anticipated complications or the warning signs, that need prompt surgical review at an appropriate level, will prevent delay in the identification of deterioration, especially if on ICU.

When you are asked to assess the postoperative patient, it is likely that they are deviating from their predicted course. From your knowledge of the pre-operative presentation, such as the examples in Table 10.1, you should have suspicions of potential complications. However, you must always use the CCrISP system of assessment to guide your management and prevent omissions. Even if you are unsure of the cause, the system will enable you to recognise whether the patient is unstable and/or deteriorating, and that the patient may require senior surgical or ICU assessment. Call for help early, but continue your systematic process of assessment and resuscitation.

## ANTICIPATING A NEED FOR ICU

You know that some patients are planned for ICU pre-operatively because of factors that predict a likely need for more intensive support, such as:

- their age
- critical nature of their diagnosis
- pre-operative co-morbidity
- acute physiological stress.

These prophylactic transfers to a higher level of monitoring allow for early recognition of any complication and so minimise the delay in treatment. Likewise, any of these factors in a deteriorating surgical patient on the ward should prompt earlier transfer to ICU.

## RECOGNISING DETERIORATION ON ICU

The benefit of more intensive monitoring is the early recognition of systemic changes since these, rather than the examination of the abdomen or chest, are far more accurate signs of deterioration. A colonic anastomotic leak should cause peritonism and distension but, if a patient is still paralysed and ventilated, these will be masked. It is more likely that subtle physiological changes such as

increasing oxygen or ventilatory requirement will raise a suspicion in such patients.

While the abdomen may seem a likely source when deterioration occurs after laparotomy, consider alternative causes such as sepsis from lines, urine or chest, or limb ischaemia in a prothrombotic state.

However, remember that, once on ICU, the patient has little physiological reserve and a missed intra-abdominal sepsis or ischaemia is often fatal!

## ASSESSING THE ABDOMEN ON ICU

### PRACTICE POINT

*Consider previous ICU patients you have seen with abdominal pathology. Were there obvious abdominal signs or did you rely on the charts to identify clinical deterioration?*

Often clinical signs on the ventilated patient can be very subtle and even misleading. It is easy to be lured into a false sense of security because the abdomen feels soft and non-distended. The charts will guide you towards recognising the problem. It may be a gradual increase in oxygen or ventilatory requirements, or an increasing dependence in inotropes to maintain perfusion. The urine output may be gradually diminishing despite adequate fluid filling.

### PRACTICE POINT

*Think of patients you have seen that have demonstrated these features. Was there a concern about re-operating, or a delay in return to theatre?*

## TABLE 10.2

### WARNING SIGNS OF SIGNIFICANT PATHOLOGY

| Warning sign | Underlying cause |
| --- | --- |
| Neutropenia (WCC < 2000 x $10^9$/l) | Overwhelming sepsis/profoundly impaired host response |
| Grossly elevated WCC (> 20,000–25,000 x $10^9$/l) | Sign of infarction<br>Also occurs post splenectomy<br>Consider *Clostridium* spp. infection if associated diarrhoea |
| Metabolic acidosis | Tissue hypoperfusion from ischaemia or sepsis |

Often, due to the subtle and gradual clinical deterioration, there are delays in taking patients to theatre. While it may be the systemic signs that herald the patient's deterioration, the diagnostic question is whether this is due to bleeding, perforation, mesenteric ischaemia, pancreatitis or sepsis and where the source may be. Within the abdomen there may be temptation to confirm the diagnosis with imaging, but one should carefully appraise the benefits of this as opposed to direct intervention with a laparotomy. In the case of a suspected colonic anastomotic leak, a CT scan and contrast enema are complementary, with the former the investigation of choice with the possibility of additional percutaneous drainage. However, a negative scan does not exclude a leak completely and the time and delays of the transfer to and from the CT scanner should be considered against the benefit of rapid drainage from an immediate return to theatre. Likewise, an ultrasound may show free fluid but that will very rarely change your management. Simple blood tests, particularly the white cell count and blood gases, may guide you towards a specific cause of deterioration as shown in Table 10.2. You should also remember to take all possible cultures (blood, pus, urine or sputum, etc.) in order to direct therapy in the longer term. If you are not sure, seek senior help and advice. Don't just organise more tests!

In more subtle postoperative changes, contrast CT arterial imaging may exclude an ischaemic cause. Isolating a focus of infection may require a labelled leukocyte scan. However, in acute deterioration there is not the time to delay and a laparotomy may be indicated.

Occasionally, negative laparotomies are performed as part of a diagnostic process when faced with a deteriorating surgical patient. This is not necessarily a wrong course of action, but extended delay of the patient who does need to return to theatre will invariably lead to a worse outcome.

## CASE SCENARIO 10.1

You are asked to assess a 45-year-old, 120 kg man on the ICU who is 10 h postoperative from a laparotomy for blunt abdominal trauma. There is concern that, despite fluid resuscitation, he remains tachycardic and hypotensive. He is still ventilated. You arrive on the ICU and the nurse asks: 'Do you think he could be bleeding?'

### HOW WOULD YOU MANAGE THIS SITUATION?

This is for you a difficult and complex assessment, especially since the patient remains ventilated. However, if you follow the CCrISP system, this patient can be assessed thoroughly and systematically in a similar manner to the non-ventilated patient (Fig. 10.1). You follow the system and your immediate management is as follows:

- A: intubated and ventilated
- B: ICU report increasing airway pressure required to ventilate
- C: P = 120 bpm, BP = 90/60 mmHg, CVP = 12 cmH$_2$O, though cardiac output is reducing. No external signs of continued haemorrhage. Minimal reduction in Hb from 9.5 to 8.6 g/dl in the last 5 h though has had 4 unit transfusion since theatre. Urine output 200 ml in the last 7 h
- D: pupils respond appropriately. Patient is paralysed
- E: this patient is obese but you note that the abdomen appears distended.

### IS THIS PATIENT STABLE OR UNSTABLE AND WHAT WOULD YOU DO AT THIS STAGE?

The patient is clearly unstable. You need to consider whether more resuscitation is required or whether to call the surgical consultant for an immediate return to theatre. It is probably reasonable to gather more information at this stage and continue with the system of assessment while the ICU staff continue resuscitation. Using the CCrISP system, you would perform a full patient assessment. The available results are (all conventional units): Hb 8.6, WCC 18.9, platelets 65, amylase 240, sodium 128, potassium 5.9, urea 12.5, pH 7.3, PO$_2$ 8.5 kPa, PaCO$_2$ 6 kPa, BE −7 (increased from −3 in last 3 h).

Chart review: the operation note reports the need for a splenectomy and extensive bleeding from the vena cava (Fig. 10.2).

### DOES THIS HELP YOU MAKE A DECISION? DO YOU HAVE A DIAGNOSIS? CONSIDER WHAT YOUR MANAGEMENT PLAN WOULD BE AND WHETHER YOU NEED ANY OTHER INVESTIGATIONS.

You should have recognised that the intra-abdominal pressure was elevated at the time of closure and simple investigation is to repeat the bladder pressure, which is now 28 mmHg. Therefore, this patient has abdominal compartment syndrome and requires immediate return to theatre to re-open his abdomen. Further delay increases the risk of worsening organ dysfunction and further resuscitation or conservative measures will be futile without immediate decompression. You arrange for the patient to return to theatre and inform the surgical consultant. On laparotomy, there is no ongoing haemorrhage and his colon is viable so the abdomen is left open as a laparostomy.

**CONSIDER THE PROBLEMS THAT MIGHT BE ENCOUNTERED WHEN THE PATIENT IS TRANSFERRED BACK TO ICU.**

## LEARNING POINT

Abdominal compartment syndrome can lead rapidly to multiple organ failure which, without immediate decompression, is invariably fatal.

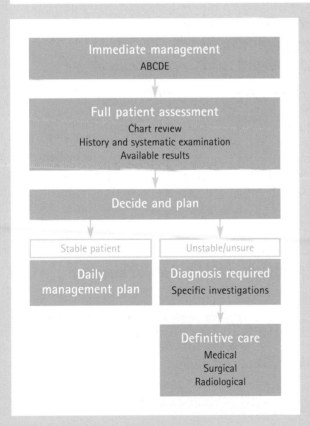

Figure 10.1 The CCrISP system of assessment.

2am    10/07/10
LAPAROTOMY FOR BLUNT TRAUMA
SPLENECTOMY. REPAIR OF GASTRIC AND CAVAL LACERATIONS
SURGEON - MR Meanor/MR. R.S. Cue
ANAESTHETIST - DR. Gas
FINDINGS - Lacerated spleen, Anterior Gastric wall laceration
and midline retroperitoneal Haematoma.
PROCEDURE - Splenectomy with individual ligation of splenic vessels
2/0 PDS repair to gastric wall.
Exploration of Haematoma, massive blood loss.
Vascular surgery called.
At least 5 litre reported blood loss
Caval and iliac venous control by compression
3/0 prolene repair to large IVC defect with impingement of
proximal R iliac vein.
No arterial injury. R. Ureter intac

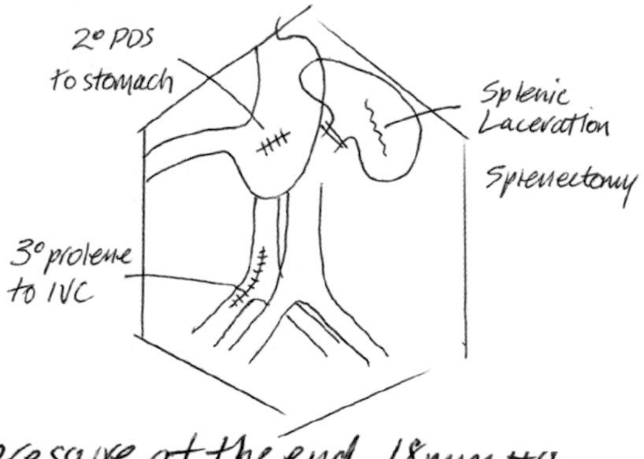

2° PDS
to stomach

Splenic
Laceration

Splenectomy

3° prolene
to IVC

Closure difficult. Intravesical pressure at the end 18mm Hg.
Post op:
    - Remain intubated.           - ICU support
    - NG Aspirate                 - Transfuse to Hb of 9g/dl
    - Massive blood loss so correct coagulopathy
    TED stockings

Figure 10.2 Operation note.

## TABLE 10.3

### SYSTEMIC EFFECTS OF ABDOMINAL COMPARTMENT SYNDROME

| System | Intra-abdominal pressure | | |
|---|---|---|---|
| | 10–15 mmHg | 16–25 mmHg | > 25 mmHg |
| Cardiovascular | | Reduced preload and increased afterload Reduced cardiac output | Reduced contractility Gross reduction in cardiac output |
| Renal | | Oliguria | Anuria |
| Gastrointestinal | Slight intestinal and hepatic ischaemia | Marked intestinal and hepatic ischaemia | Bowel infarction Hepatic failure |
| CNS | | Minimal effect | Increased intracranial pressure |

## SPECIFIC SURGICAL SITE COMPLICATIONS

### ABDOMINAL COMPARTMENT SYNDROME

Abdominal compartment syndrome or the presence of elevated intra-abdominal pressure is a significant cause of morbidity and mortality among critically ill surgical and medical patients. As shown in Table 10.3, significant systemic effects occur with a rise in abdominal pressure.

The actual development of intra-abdominal hypertension (IAH) is a continuum of pathophysiological changes that begins with a disturbance of regional blood flow and culminates in frank end-organ failure, due to the development of abdominal compartment syndrome. The aetiology of IAH may be intra-abdominal, particularly in abdominal trauma patients (see scenario above), pancreatitis or following aortic surgery, but can also occur due to an extra-abdominal cause, such as burns or sepsis associated with aggressive fluid resuscitation.

The intra-abdominal pressure is expressed in mmHg, with the usual level being sub-atmospheric to 0 mmHg, though elevation to the range of 5–7 mmHg is common.

IAH is defined as a sustained or repeated elevation of IAP > 12 mmHg and is graded as: I, 12–15 mmHg; II, 16–20 mmHg; III, 21–25 mmHg; IV > 25 mmHg. Grade IV requires surgical decompression.

The cardiac effect of IAH is due to elevation of the diaphragm and the subsequent rise in intrathoracic pressure, which in turn reduces the venous return and cardiac output. Such changes are far more likely in the hypotensive patient and so early signs of pressure elevation should be managed by fluid resuscitation.

Intra-abdominal pressure is measured by assessing intravesicular/bladder pressure. The measurement should occur at the end of expiration with the patient in the complete supine position, after ensuring that abdominal muscle contractions are absent. The transducer is zeroed at the level of the mid axilliary line and connected to the bladder catheter. Sterile saline (25 ml) is inserted into the bladder to act as a conductive fluid column.

Abdominal compartment syndrome is the progression of pressure induced end-organ changes and, if due to intra-abdominal causes such as trauma or acute pancreatitis, is characterised by rapid deterioration which if not recognised and treated is commonly fatal.

The expedient treatment of ACS is to re-open or perform a laparotomy wound in order to decompress the abdomen. As in the scenario above, a thorough wash-out of all fluid/blood should be performed, with a detailed inspection for sites of bleeding. The bowel should be carefully inspected for signs of ischaemia.

There are a number of options available at the end of the laparotomy though, almost invariably, primary closure should not be considered. A large saline infusion bag can be opened up and sutured to the fascial edges in order to provide a temporary seal of the abdominal cavity. Specific bowel bags can also be used in a similar way. This may later be converted to a mesh covered with packs or a negative pressure dressing. There is some concern that negative pressure can encourage the formation of a fistula from oedematous and friable bowel. Fig. 10.3 shows a laparostomy in a patient who later underwent successful split skin graft closure.

Postoperatively, laparostomy patients can be challenging for ICU staff to manage, particularly from the nursing point of view. The surgical staff should liaise closely with the ICU staff and predict problems with fluid and temperature losses through the laparostomy wound, the potential for sepsis especially with respect to any underlying vascular grafts, and make a plan to achieve wound closure.

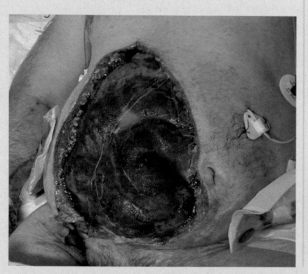
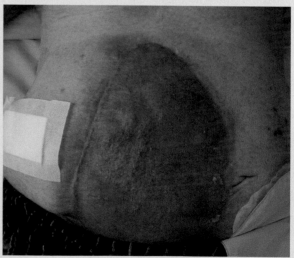

Figure 10.3 A laparostomy and outcome following mesh closure and skin graft.

## CASE SCENARIO 10.2

You are asked by the ICU staff to assess a 25-year-old man who, 14 h following laparotomy for a penetrating abdominal stab wound, is becoming increasingly unstable with a BE of −8. You follow the CCrISP system to assess and resuscitate the patient systematically. Your findings from the initial management are:

- A: intubated
- B: ventilated
- C: P = 120 bpm; BP = 95/75; CVP = 6 cmH$_2$O, cold peripheries, pedal pulses not palpable, requiring increasing dose of noradrenaline, urine output 250 ml since return from theatre
- D: pupils respond appropriately. Patient is paralysed
- E: abdominal wound is laparostomy, with appearance of right-sided stoma.

Full patient assessment of available results: Hb 9.0, WCC 24, platelets 75, amylase 200, sodium 130, potassium 6.5, urea 16, pH 7.2, PO$_2$ 18.5 kPa, PaCO$_2$ 5 kPa, BE −8, lactate 5, CK 4000 u/l. Chart review showed the patient was stabbed in the abdomen after an evening out drinking and suffered significant blood loss at the scene. He had a systolic pressure of only 70 mmHg on arrival in A&E. He was immediately taken to theatre, where laparotomy findings were a distal aortic laceration and a small sigmoid laceration with minimal contamination. The sigmoid laceration was closed primarily but defunctioning ileostomy performed. Significant blood loss occurred before and during the aortic repair with repeated episodes of clamping. It was a long procedure; therefore, abdominal packing was inserted with a re-look planned at 24 h.

### WHAT DO YOU THINK MIGHT ACCOUNT FOR THE DETERIORATION AND HOW WOULD YOU MANAGE THE SITUATION?

It is unlikely to be abdominal compartment syndrome because of the laparostomy. You need to perform a thorough systematic examination, in particular looking at his lower limb vasculature because of the history of aortic injury. Only femoral pulses are palpable; both feet are cold and poorly perfused. From toes to knees, the calves are very swollen and tense. The patient is clearly unstable and requires no further investigations to confirm the diagnosis of bilateral lower limb compartment syndrome. Arrangements are made for urgent fasciotomies to be performed. Upon performing the fasciotomies, all muscle groups are very oedematous and immediately bulge from the wounds. Some areas of muscle do not contract to electrical (diathermy) or physical stimuli, though other areas contract normally.

## LOWER LIMB COMPARTMENT SYNDROME

Limb compartment syndrome should always be considered when there has been a period of ischaemia and perfusion. Case Scenario 10.2 highlights the need for thorough systematic assessment and prompt therapeutic action. A delay in recognising limb compartment syndrome can rapidly lead to irreversible muscle damage resulting in permanent neuromuscular defects within 12 hours. This may necessitate amputations. Also, aggressive fluid resuscitation is required to minimise the effects of myoglobin from muscle breakdown that can cause renal failure.

Lower limb trauma and associated hypotension may lead to re-perfusion with significant rises in interstitial pressure and subsequent compartment syndrome. Beware also a prolonged operation in the lithotomy position; this can also produce compartment syndrome and, any delay in treatment, minimises the chances of limb salvage. If there was any doubt in the diagnosis, compartment pressures can be performed with a needle inserted into each compartment, with the knowledge that tissue necrosis can occur with an interstitial pressure as low as 30 mmHg.

### PRACTICE POINT

*An old surgical word-of-mouth adage is that if you are thinking of the need for fasciotomies, then you should perform them without further discussion!*

## COMPARTMENTS TO DECOMPRESS

The lateral compartment/superficial posterior/deep posterior and anterior compartments of the leg all require decompression and this should be performed in a sterile environment in theatre.

After the procedure there will, due to the muscle oedema, be a lot of fluid discharge from the wounds. It is important that instructions for dressing are clear and that no compression should be applied to reduce blood or fluid loss from the wounds. Occasionally, brisk venous bleeding can occur from the wounds that may require further surgical exploration to control the source.

Compartment syndrome can also occur in the thigh and upper limb and the management principles are identical.

## BURST ABDOMEN

This complication is at the other end of the spectrum from compartment syndrome though the immediate management is similar to a laparostomy with the aim to keep the exposed viscera warm and moist and minimise the loss of fluid and temperature. It now occurs rarely, since the advent of mass closure with synthetic monofilament sutures. When it does occur, the 'pink sign', of serosanguinous discharge some 8–10 days after the initial surgery, usually heralds it. If there were little systemic upset, the abdomen should be resutured within 3–4 hours; however, if there is systemic instability, it would be better to manage the wound as a laparostomy temporarily.

## POSTOPERATIVE BLEEDING

Despite anticipating bleeding problems, postoperative haemorrhage can be covert with the only signs manifesting in progressive haemodynamic deterioration. An example would be after an angiogram with a high puncture of the common femoral artery, when a retroperitoneal bleed is not uncommon. The ability to predict this complication should be high, providing the ability to react early with surgical correction.

Primary haemorrhage occurs at the time of surgery. If difficult to control – particularly if from the liver, pelvis or other inaccessible sites – consideration should be given to packing the effected area with a view to return to theatre at 48 hours for removal of packs and re-inspection of the operative site.

A reactive haemorrhage is generally due to a technical failure such as a slipped ligature, which may present itself while the patient is in recovery or having returned to the ward from theatre.

Again, this requires a thorough systematic assessment to ensure prompt detection and return to theatre. Examples where this might occur include after splenectomy due to a short gastric ligature coming loose. Even though the vessels are small, this bleed can still cause a rapid deterioration and cardiovascular compromise. Reactive haemorrhage may also occur after fluid resuscitation in trauma patients when the increased perfusion pressure may initiate bleeding.

## CASE SCENARIO 10.2 CONTINUED

You are asked to re-assess the patient from Case Scenario 10.2, 4 h after the returning to ICU, with blood staining of the laparostomy bag and a 2.5 g/dl fall in Hb (now 6.5 g/dl compared to 9 g/dl at the time of leaving theatre).

### HOW WOULD YOU MANAGE THIS SITUATION?

This is often a difficult balance between a decision to return to theatre and control of coagulopathy. This decision should be made in collaboration with the ICU staff. There are a number of factors that will predispose to coagulopathy, including the massive blood transfusion, hypothermia and reperfusion injury.

### LEARNING POINT

A coagulopathy is common in critically ill patients and should be considered as a cause of any overt or concealed haemorrhage. Any clotting problem should ideally be corrected prior to re-operation, and this may require close collaboration between surgeon, anaesthetist and haematology staff. Be careful not to ascribe surgical bleeding to a general bleed associated with a minor coagulopathy, as trying to correct the clotting will not improve the situation. Indeed, further delay may cause worsening of the coagulopathy and a cycle of deterioration. It is better to control the specific source and correct the coagulopathy in theatre.

Other factors to consider with generalised bleeding problems are:
- effect of anticoagulant therapy
- a recent large transfusion
- the presence of sepsis or DIC
- previously unrecognised concomitant bleeding disorders, either congenital (e.g. Waldenström's macroglobulinaemia) or acquired e.g. drugs).

Secondary haemorrhage occurs much later, often 7–8 days following a procedure. It is often related to infective complications but still may be unexpected and unheralded; control may be difficult to achieve. More proximal vascular control is often required and should be considered at the time of re-operation.

---

### PRACTICE POINT

*Reversing a coagulopathy will not stop surgical bleeding. Correct the coagulopathy while addressing the source of the bleeding.*

---

### NECROTISING FASCIITIS

Necrotising infection can be difficult to diagnose; early diagnosis and targeted treatment is essential. Any diagnostic delay increases the mortality, which has a range of 25–73%. Immunocompromised patients on chemotherapy or steroids are vulnerable, but diabetes is the leading predisposing factor. The causative bacteria are synergistic and cause an infection involving the subcutaneous fascial layer, inducing extensive undermining of surrounding tissues. Presentation may be primary, where no portal of entry or causative factor is found, or secondary, due to a precipitating event such as a peri-anal abscess.

The initial features may be subtle including influenza-like symptoms and localised discomfort or pain. Subsequently, the limb or painful area begins to swell and may show a purplish rash. The skin marking will then blister with blackish

fluid, and patients undergo severe systemic collapse due to sepsis. The treatment required is prompt, aggressive debridement, with wide excision of all involved tissue back to bleeding edges. This may be quite extensive, and can take more than one operation. Patients usually require systemic support along with broad-spectrum antibiotics.

### ANASTOMOTIC LEAKAGE

The typical signs of anastomotic leakage are of systemic instability with abdominal pain and/or rigid abdomen, tachycardia and fever. However, there may be a far more insidious presentation with low-grade fever, a prolonged ileus or failure to thrive. Therefore, anastomotic leakage should be considered as a cause for any unexplained postoperative deterioration following bowel surgery. This is particularly the case for laparoscopic colonic surgery, where there may be a reluctance to re-operate on vague clinical signs. Leak rates for laparoscopic colonic surgery range from 2.5–12% in the literature. While less likely, it should be recognised that a defunctioning stoma does not exclude the possibility of an anastomotic leak.

In trying to anticipate anastomotic leakage, it is important to review the notes and the charts. For example, does the anaesthetic chart indicate pre-operative dehydration or any episodes of peri-operative hypotension? Does the operation note comment on the quality of perfusion in the mesenteric vessels? In an emergency case, does the ICU chart show that inotropes were required, that may have caused mesenteric vasoconstriction? Factors that predispose to leak are shown in Table 10.4.

| TABLE 10.4 |
| --- |

**RISK FACTORS FOR INTESTINAL ANASTOMOTIC LEAKAGE**

**Anastomotic technique**
- Tension, poor anatomical blood supply (particularly after anterior resection), unrecognised mesenteric vessel damage, poor suture technique (eversion or mismatch)

**Local factors**
- Obstruction, ischaemia or peritonitis

**Systemic factors**
- Shock (excessive bowel preparation or excessive blood loss), age, malnutrition, immunosuppression

| TABLE 10.5 |
| --- |

**PRINCIPLES OF RE-OPERATIVE SURGERY FOR ABDOMINAL SEPSIS**

- Prepare the patient as well as is reasonably possible
- Anticipate the difficulty of re-operative surgery and involve a senior surgeon
- Aim to deal with the source of the primary problem definitively
- Exteriorise leaking bowel
- Remove dead tissue
- Culture pus and drain sepsis
- Consider gastrostomy or jejunostomy for ease of future management

In trying to make the diagnosis of a leak, a CT scan and contrast enema may have a complementary role, though the CT scan with contrast is the likely radiological procedure of choice. If a collection is shown to indicate a localised leak, a CT- or ultrasound-guided drainage may be indicated. However, major leakage has a significant mortality (10–15%) and so prompt re-operation is indicated with exteriorisation of suitable ends of small and large bowel. At this time, the need for nutritional support and the potential routes of access should be considered.

It is important to anticipate the difficulty of re-operative surgery on ICU patients and follow the principles shown in Table 10.5. A senior surgeon should be involved early in the decision making, and certainly in the surgery.

## THE MANAGEMENT OF INTESTINAL FISTULAE

The evolution of an abdominal wall intestinal fistula provides significant management challenges, which are likely to require high dependency care even if there is no complicating infection or sepsis. The management involves the monitoring of significant fluid and electrolyte losses and their subsequent replacement along with nutritional therapy. Also involved is the physical management of the fistula; the surrounding skin requires protection by dressings or bags, and this will require the input of the stoma therapist.

When a fistula occurs postoperatively, assess by the CCrISP protocol and then utilise the 'SNAP' (sepsis, nutrition, anatomy, procedure) protocol.

| S | Sepsis | Obtain adequate drainage |
|---|---|---|
| | | May involve CT-guided or surgical drainage |
| | | May involve defunctioning of the bowel |
| N | Nutrition | Provide nutritional support |
| | | Often this will be parenteral |
| A | Anatomy | Delineate using imaging the site of leak |
| | | CT with contrast is preferred choice |
| P | Procedure | Ultimately aim for reparative procedure |
| | | Delay until patient is well enough to predict success (this may be months) |

## CASE SCENARIO 10.3

Consider the surgical case from Case Scenario 10.1, in which the patient developed a compartment syndrome and required an urgent laparotomy. The abdomen was washed out and closed primarily at 48 h with a large bore drain inserted via the left iliac fossa along the paracolic gutter into the splenic bed. The drain produces 50 ml of haemoserous fluid for 48 h; however, before it can be removed, suddenly drains 300 ml of similar fluid.

### HOW WOULD YOU MANAGE THE PATIENT? COULD THIS BE A FISTULA AND IF SO WHAT IS THE POTENTIAL SOURCE?

As always, use the CCrISP system with simultaneous assessment and resuscitation. Following immediate management, you decide that the patient is stable and proceed to the full patient assessment. On review of the operation note, you should note the gastric repair and the splenectomy, and consider a missed injury to the pancreas or small bowel, or a leak from the gastric repair.

A pancreatic fistula (remember to send the draining fluid for an amylase level) may give further problems due to the digestive actions of the pancreatic fluid, with concern for the various sites of surgical repair. A high small bowel fistula can cause high volume losses of fluids and electrolytes and rapid changes to acid–base balance. These are complex problems and it is important to recognise them early. A diagnosis is essential and, while testing the fluid for amylase may suggest a pancreatic fistula, further radiological investigation is likely to be required, including contrast-enhanced CT. Having made a diagnosis, the SNAP protocol should be used to manage the patient further. Specialist, senior help should be enlisted for the management of intestinal fistulae.

# MANAGEMENT OF STOMAS AND DRAINS

There are various stomas that may form a part of the postoperative management of patients. Both on the ward and critical care areas, this should be directed by the surgical team with the support of the stoma care nurse, or nutritional support team in the case of feeding stomas.

## FEEDING GASTROSTOMY OR JEJUNOSTOMY

The timing, content and volume of nutritional support should be planned according to bowel function with the surgical team liaising with the dietician or nutritional support team (see Chapter 13).

There must be clear advice given on timing of removal and obvious marking of the feeding stoma to prevent accidental removal if mistaken for a drain. Ten days is usually the minimum time allowed for a suitable seal to form.

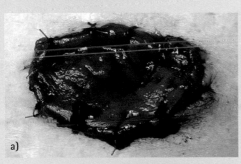

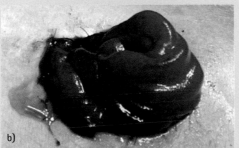

Figure 10.4 a) End colostomy, and b) loop ileostomy.

## FAECAL STOMAS

These may be temporary, loop or end type as shown in Fig. 10.4; their appearances are different, as are the difficulties in their management.

Small bowel effluent from an ileostomy will irritate the skin and so the stoma is formed as a spout, whereas a colostomy will be flush to the skin since the effluent is more solid and less irritant. If a bridge is used for a loop stoma, the operation notes should be very clear as to how long it should remain.

Irrespective of type, if there is concern with respect to the stoma's condition or function it should be inspected, which will require:

- Removal of the stoma bag
- Assessment of the colour/perfusion of the stoma and the contents of the bag (is the stoma actually functioning? Is there any blood to indicate more proximal bleeding?)
- Assessment of the skin around the stoma (is there cellulitis or separation of the stoma from the skin? Is the stoma in close proximity to wound giving risk of contamination?)
- Digital examination of the stoma (and the requirement for direct observation with a proctoscope to determine the extent of any discolouration).

Remember that while a complication of the stoma may lead to systemic deterioration, conversely systemic deterioration can lead to stoma deterioration.

The small bowel effluent from an ileostomy is usually 500–700 ml/day but, initially, on starting to function these volumes may be much greater requiring careful electrolyte monitoring and replacement.

It is important to involve a stoma therapist as early as possible, especially with respect to skin protection. The therapist also provides vital psychological support to the patients with a stoma and, if possible, this meeting should occur pre-operatively with marking of potential stoma sites.

## MANAGEMENT OF SURGICAL DRAINS

There is a continued debate as to the value and usage of drains; nevertheless, their presence in the critically ill surgical patient requires them to be assessed and managed effectively and appropriately.

Within the assessment of the surgical patient, the amount and type of drainage, and whether that is expected, should be determined and documented. The drain site should be inspected and notes reviewed to determine the nature and positioning of drains, and the rationale for placement. Drains should be clearly marked if there is more that one and it is the surgeon's responsibility to state when they should be removed.

## POST-SURGICAL WOUND MANAGEMENT

Surgical wound infections are a common hospital acquired infection (~12%) and are subsequently an important cause of morbidity and mortality. Therefore, their prevention should be a primary management objective. The risk of infection should relate to whether the surgery was clean, clean with risk of contamination or contaminated. It should not be a marker of hospital staff hygiene! Remember to ensure good hand-washing before and after the assessment of wounds to diminish the risk of direct contamination.

A wound can be contaminated with bacteria without a host response and then deemed to be colonised when the bacteria multiply and initiate a host response. When this bacterial multiplication causes a delay in wound healing, the colonisation is critical and is usually associated with wound pain. Once there is both a delay in healing and an associated host response the wound is infected. By using the CCrISP method of assessment, all wounds should have a postoperative plan with observation for the early signs of infection of redness, swelling, heat and pain. Dependent on peri-operative risk and/or the potential consequences of infection, the patient may have had prophylactic antibiotics and this and any postoperative regimen should be clear from a review of the charts. The majority of wounds are closed primarily; however, if there is local wound deterioration, it may be that the sutures should be removed to allow drainage or antibiotic treatment may suffice. The timings of suture removal are a surgical decision and, especially on ICU, should be clearly documented within any surgical management plan.

## SUMMARY

While it is sometimes difficult to assess the post-surgical patient, particularly on the ICU, the CCrISP process allows a structured assessment that will highlight the likely cause of any deterioration. By assessing the risk factors, many surgical-site complications can be anticipated or recognised early. Thus, postoperative management plans should highlight which signs require early surgical review, such as the increasing abdominal pressure that would trigger the conversion to a laparostomy.

There will always be surgical complications but the risk should be minimised and problems should be recognised and managed promptly and effectively.

# 11

## Fluid and electrolyte management

## OBJECTIVES

This chapter will help you to:

- be better able to manage complex fluid balance in critically ill patients
- be aware of common pitfalls in fluid management in surgical patients
- understand better water and electrolyte balance in the critically ill
- be aware of common electrolyte abnormalities and their causes and management
- understand the properties of common intravenous fluids.

Assessing fluid balance and prescribing appropriate fluid is an important daily task for surgeons; as the registrar, it will be often be your responsibility to ensure that this is carried out safely and accurately. In many surgical patients, the process becomes potentially complex because of multiple sources of fluid loss and several types of fluid input. However, with a logical approach and a clear understanding of a few basics, even complex cases can be dealt with. Conversely, poor prescribing remains a common cause of avoidable morbidity and mortality, either from inadequate resuscitation of the critically ill or excessive provision of fluids to elective patients.

## PATIENT GROUPS

Patients are all different. Fluid needs are determined by baseline needs (dependent, in turn, on BMI), pre-existing fluid deficits and on going abnormal losses. However, in major surgical practice, we see two differing groups of patients who handle fluids differently. Obviously, patients may switch between groups if complications develop.

### CRITICAL ILLNESS AND EMERGENCY SURGERY

In critical illness and after complicated major surgery, the obligatory extracellular volume required to maintain adequate venous return to the heart rises due to the loss of salt water and protein into sites of tissue damage, obstructed bowel, serous body cavities and the relaxation of the peripheral vascular bed. In some situations (*e.g.* sepsis), the amount of sequestered fluid may be prodigious due to an enormous capillary leak and sufficient to cause circulatory failure. This is the situation seen often in critically ill surgical patients. Consequently, it is reasonable to suspect hypovolaemia in most patients and act accordingly.

Epidural anaesthesia causes vasodilatation and this increased vascular space needs filling or controlling. This is particularly so if the patient has also been cold after surgery and vasodilates further as they warm up. In these patients, the commonest error is inadequate fluid resuscitation, whether in volume, fluid type or rate of delivery.

## UNCOMPLICATED ELECTIVE SURGERY

By way of contrast, major but uncomplicated surgery produces a different situation. Surgery itself causes activation of the anti-diuretic hormone (ADH) and angiotensin-aldosterone, thereby retaining fluids and causing reduced urine output for 24–48 hours. Thus, in a well patient with otherwise normal parameters, isolated, modest oliguria can be acceptable. With fast-track recovery programmes advocating early and liberal oral intake and less in the way of bowel preparation (which dehydrates the patient significantly), the elective patient is less likely to be volume depleted. These patients often need much less in the way of postoperative fluids; in these 'well' patients, excessive fluids cause more harm than good. Here, excessive provision of sodium and water is now recognised as the principal cause of avoidable problems. This is a very different set of circumstances to the critically ill patient who, not infrequently, needs intravenous fluids rapidly for life-saving resuscitation. Fluid resuscitation from shock using an appropriate colloid or crystalloid was dealt with in the chapters on assessment and shock (Chapters 2 and 8).

## CLINICAL ASSESSMENT

The patient should be fully assessed according to the CCrISP system. Take particular note of indices of volume status and perfusion, including vital signs, CVP/JVP, skin perfusion and turgor and oedema (which appears on the sacrum if bed-bound). Note the patient's underlying age, BMI, general condition, operative treatment and timing, co-morbid diseases and drugs.

Along with clinical examination, the fluid balance chart is the principal mechanism of assessment; however, accuracy of fluid balance charts is variable and, with experience, one learns which ward's charts can be relied upon the most! Insensible loss increases markedly with fever, respiratory rate and the breathing of dry $O_2$ – all of which can apply in the day or two after major surgery. As much as 500–1000 ml can be lost daily.

There is no one formula that can be applied to all situations and regular frequent clinical assessment of the patient will be required to adjust the content and volumes of fluid replacement. This should be done at least daily, more often in the unstable. Occasionally with chronic overload, daily weighing of the patient, when feasible, can be of assistance and complements the fluid balance chart.

## FLUID COMPARTMENTS AND CONTROL OF VOLUME

The total body water volume (~45 l) is distributed through the intracellular and extravascular compartments in a ratio of 2:1 (Fig. 11.1).

The total volume of water is controlled by both central osmoreceptors and volume receptors that affect thirst and the release of ADH. Volume receptors will release ADH even in the face of hyponatraemia and a low plasma osmolality. Extracellular fluid (ECF) volume (of which blood volume is a special part) is maintained by the presence of sodium and its accompanying anions which are largely excluded from the intracellular compartment by the action of the Na/K pump. The body responds rapidly to a fall in central volume or renal perfusion by reducing renal sodium excretion to extremely low levels. Thus, there are two mechanisms for retaining water or sodium

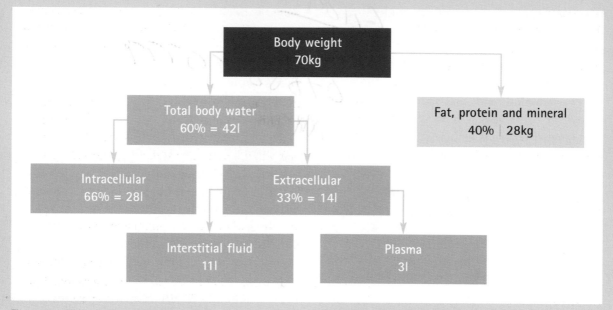

Figure 11.1 **Fluid distribution in the body.**

rapidly. On the other hand, excretion is more passive and often slower, so the response to surgical stress favours fluid retention and overload. In critical illness this has some advantages, as many of the effects of surgery cause fluid loss. When assessing patients, consider:

- assessment of fluid and electrolyte status requires both clinical and biochemical examination
- intracellular volume is extremely difficult to assess clinically
- the extracellular compartment is easier to assess clinically as increased salt and water manifests itself as oedema and salt and water depletion by effects on the circulation
- the balance between blood volume and ECF is maintained by the oncotic pressure and the relative leakiness of the capillaries

- in haemorrhage, the plasma volume is partly replenished from the ECF
- in sepsis, gross capillary leak and a low oncotic pressure contribute to oedema and hypovolaemia.

## BIOCHEMICAL ASSESSMENT

This clinical re-assessment is assisted by biochemical measurement, primarily of blood but also, on occasion, of urine and other fluid being lost from the body (*e.g.* fistula fluid).

### WATER

Patients usually need 1500–2000 ml water daily, depending on weight and fluid status. The basal water requirement is 30-40ml/kg/day.

## SODIUM

Normal basal requirements for sodium are 50–100 mmol/day but this can vary a lot with surgical illness. Drug solutions can contain significant amounts of sodium. Care must also be taken to ensure that a false value for sodium is not obtained by venepuncture from a limb with a running fluid infusion or if there is frank lipaemia (*e.g.* intralipid administration).

### Hyponatraemia

Often, the serum sodium gives a clearer idea of the relative water state of the body than of sodium status, hence clinical assessment is essential. A patient with hyponatraemia of, for example, 125 mmol/l may be sodium depleted (hypovolaemic), sodium replete or sodium overloaded (oedematous due to cardiac, renal or hepatic disease) depending upon the relative quantity of water in the extra-cellular space (Table 11.1). Dilutional hyponatraemia from excessive infusion of water (as 5% dextrose) is still seen on surgical wards.

The management of hyponatraemia may be rapid sodium chloride infusion, water restriction or diuretic plus water restriction depending upon clinical assessment of volume status. Remember that water cannot be excreted by the kidney in the presence of extracellular fluid depletion (see above – primacy of volume) and that the syndrome of 'inappropriate ADH secretion' can only be diagnosed once the patient has been shown to be in sodium balance.

Correction of hyponatraemia should be achieved at a similar rate to that at which it developed to avoid cerebral fluid shifts. Given normal renal

**TABLE 11.1**

HYPONATRAEMIA – TYPES AND CAUSES

| | ECF volume | ECF volume | ECF volume |
|---|---|---|---|
| | Low | Normal/slightly raised | High |
| | (NaCl ---, H$_2$O -) | (NaCl normal, H$_2$O +) | (NaCl +, H$_2$O +++) |
| **Urine Na high** (> 20 mmol/l) | Diuretics (excessive) Salt losing renal disease Mineralocorticoid deficiency | Glucocorticoid deficiency Hypothyroidism SIADH | Renal failure |
| **Urine Na low** (< 20 mmol/l) | Extrarenal loss: (i) Outwith body | (ii) Sequestration | Dilutional (i.v. 5% dextrose) Cirrhosis Cardiac failure Nephrotic syndrome |

function, water overload can be cleared by the administration of diuretic and 0.9% sodium chloride to replace the fluid excreted by the kidney. Hypertonic saline is seldom necessary.

## Hypernatraemia

This can be caused by abnormal intake or administration of hypertonic fluid (*e.g.* 8.4% sodium bicarbonate), but is more commonly due to abnormal water loss (fever, diabetes insipidus or mellitus, osmotic diuretics) in a situation where intake of water is impaired. Correction is with water (via the gut) or by intravenous 5% dextrose.

## POTASSIUM

The usual requirement of potassium is 40–80 mmol/day.

## Hypokalaemia

Common causes of hypokalaemia in surgical practice include: (i) renal losses; (ii) intestinal losses; and (iii) medical losses (no K in the drip!).

Plasma potassium is a poor reflection of the total body potassium content as plasma contains only 1% of the body total. The rate of change of the extracellular potassium concentration is more important than the absolute value. Hypokalaemia is usually the result of loss of potassium from the body via the kidney or bowel (diuretics, tubular disease, diarrhoea or laxatives). Acute changes in plasma potassium may occur as potassium moves into cells during the correction of an acidosis, secondary to the acute release of catecholamines (cerebral bleed or trauma), administration of salbutamol or upon refeeding with the start of anabolic activity. The level should be kept above 3.5 mmol/l by stopping any avoidable losses and the administration of potassium.

## Hyperkalaemia

A rapidly rising plasma potassium level is a medical emergency and will result in respiratory muscle weakness and cardiac arrest from which it is extremely difficult to be resuscitated.

The primary route of potassium excretion is via the kidney in the distal nephron under the influence of aldosterone. Renal failure, hypoadrenalism, distal nephron disease (*e.g.* chronic obstructive nephropathy) or drugs that affect the renin–aldosterone system (*e.g.* ACE inhibitors) will all impair the excretion of potassium. Where there is a sudden movement of potassium out of cells due to trauma, drugs (suxamethonium), ischaemic/hypoxic damage or a sudden rise in hydrogen ion concentration, patients with impaired renal excretion will be particularly vulnerable.
A classical example is the hypovolaemic patient with a metabolic acidosis plus respiratory compensation who has anaesthesia induced with suxamethonium, is then underventilated with consequent sudden fall in pH and suffers a cardiac arrest shortly after induction. There is no absolute level above which the signs and symptoms appear and effects are related to the rate of rise as much as the plasma concentration. A chronic potassium level of 6.0 mmol/l will be well tolerated but may be fatal if the result of a rapid change from 4 mmol/l. Levels of this magnitude require rapid, specific treatment (see Chapter 9) plus reversal of the primary condition and removal of any precipitant drugs, if possible.

## CALCIUM

The calcium level in the plasma is normally kept within a narrow range under the influence of parathyroid hormone, 1,25-dihyroxy-vitamin $D_3$ and renal function. The active component is the ionised fraction which is unbound to albumin. Total levels have to be regarded in relation to the albumin level or the ionised fraction has to be measured directly.

### Hypercalcaemia

Severe hypercalcaemia will affect neural tissue and damage renal tubular function. In the critically ill, this is most often due to paraneoplastic hypercalcaemia. Hypercalcaemia diminishes the kidney's ability to retain salt and the resultant hypovolaemia reduces the ability of the kidney to excrete calcium. Dysrhythmias may occur. Establishing a saline diuresis will normally help reduce the level. If this fails, the administration of a bisphosphonate intravenously will reduce the level of calcium. Effective treatment of the primary cause will also bring the level back to normal. The development of hypercalcaemia in association with recurrence of a solid tumour is usually an indication of a poor prognosis.

### Hypocalcaemia

Apparent severe hypocalcaemia may be found in the critically ill if total plasma level is measured without reference to the albumin level. An absolute hypocalcaemia level is seen in acute pancreatitis, acute rhabdomyolysis and following thyroid surgery. Treatment is by the administration of calcium, treatment of the primary condition and in post parathyroidectomy syndrome or vitamin D deficiency, administration of activated vitamin D analogues. In those situations of critical illness with intact parathyroid function, aggressive administration of calcium should be limited to situations where there is clinical evidence of hypocalcaemia rather than attempting to achieve a given value.

## MAGNESIUM

Magnesium is the second most important intracellular cation after potassium. Magnesium is essential for the normal functioning of nerve and muscle. Depletion causes confusion and seizures and is associated with a range of dysrhythmias, while excess causes muscle paralysis and central nervous depression. In the critically ill, hypomagnesaemia is common in the early recovery period of severe insults such as peritonitis. Chronic losses from the bowel (diarrhoea), kidney (loop diuretics), and alcohol abuse contribute. As with potassium, plasma levels reflect total body magnesium poorly but a plasma level below 0.6 mmol/l associated with a condition likely to cause magnesium deficiency or the presence of symptoms should precipitate supplementation. This is best done intravenously in the acute stage to avoid the purgative effects of magnesium salts. The plasma level should not exceed 1.5 mmol/l. Critically ill patients with dysrhythmias should have magnesium levels checked as treatment with magnesium contributes to the control of several dysrhythmic states.

Significant hypermagnesaemia is almost always secondary to iatrogenic administration in the presence of impaired renal function (e.g. as magnesium sulphate for eclampsia).

## PHOSPHATE

Phosphate is present in any protein containing food and is absorbed from the gut. The kidney excretes phosphate under the influence of parathyroid hormone. High levels will be seen in renal impairment or following massive muscle or bowel necrosis. In the short term, this is usually not a major problem unless large quantities of calcium are administered.

Hypophosphataemia is commonly seen during recovery from critically illness: as cell function is restored, phosphate is taken back into cells with potassium and magnesium. When the phosphate level falls below 0.6 mmol/l, there are effects that can be measured regarding respiratory and other skeletal muscle function plus effects upon the functioning of the immune system. Replacement will come with feeding but, with levels below 0.6 mmol/l, intravenous supplementation will be required given slowly over 24 hours.

## TRACE METALS

There are many trace metals that are essential to normal cellular function and the healing process (*e.g.* zinc, copper and selenium). In situations where there is prolonged dependence upon parenteral feeding or prolonged gut dysfunction, consideration must be given to the measurement and necessary supplementation of their intake.

## APPROACH TO THE PRESCRIPTION OF FLUID AND ELECTROLYTES

This should be read in conjunction with the section in the chapter on nutrition (Chapter 13). In the critically ill, fluid replacement will be guided by the clinical situation, which is constantly changing. Requirements will be dependent upon many factors, but with three main headings: (i) basal requirements; (ii) existing fluid and electrolyte excess or deficit; and (iii) continuing abnormal losses.

Basal requirements (1500–2500 ml of water, 100 mmol Na and 80 mmol K) are influenced by a number of factors including body weight (Table 11.2). Age and cardiac or renal disease can jeopardise the patient's ability to correct imbalances so greater care is then needed. Intravenous fluids should be used for as short a period as possible – this is particularly so in well patients (*e.g.* after elective surgery).

Pre-existing fluid and electrolyte excess or deficit need factoring in – potassium deficit takes some time to correct, for example. Oedema takes some days to resolve, typically as the surgical patient recovers from major surgery and the epidural is removed.

Abnormal losses usually change gradually. These might include insensible loss of water dependent upon fever, continuing loss from the gastrointestinal or renal tract, or other effects of recent surgery, with fluid redistribution or loss from open wounds. As well as noting yesterday's outputs, your clinical assessment should help you predict, to some degree, how these losses might change today. For example, a patient recovering from laparotomy with a soft abdomen and now passing flatus, may be expected to tolerate more oral intake successfully. Hence previous nasogastric losses will likely resolve and need for intravenous fluid will decrease as oral intake increases. On the other hand, we need to be realistic about tolerance of oral intake in ill patients. Just because it is prescribed or permitted, does not mean it will be taken or tolerated. If, at this point, the fluid balance is no longer charted, then problems may develop.

## TABLE 11.2

### SOME CONSIDERATIONS FOR FLUID THERAPY

- Fluid isotonic for sodium will be required to maintain adequate extracellular volume.
- Water (oral or 5% dextrose) is needed to maintain intracellular volume and provide sufficient volume to excrete the renal load of solute waste.
- The volume of clear intravenous fluids will need to be reduced depending on the volume being given by other routes or forms (drugs, oral intake, nutrition, blood, etc.).
- Electrolyte deficiencies will need to be corrected as well as basal needs being met.

## TABLE 11.3

### FLUID LOSSES

**Losses that approximate extracellular fluid**
- Blood loss
- Vomiting
- Diarrhoea
- Gut fistulae
- Postoperative 'third space' sequestration
- Systemic inflammatory response syndrome (*e.g.* sepsis, burns, pancreatitis)
- Diabetes mellitus (hyperglycaemia)

**Losses that are principally water**
- Fever
- Increased respiratory rate
- Prolonged water deprivation
- Diabetes insipidus

## REPLACING ABNORMAL LOSSES

As a general rule, abnormal losses should be replaced with a fluid having the same composition as that which is being lost, and in a similar volume. However, matching the fluid exactly is not always necessary as the kidneys compensate efficiently under many circumstances.

Losses can be divided into those that consist more or less of extracellular fluid (ECF) or its equivalent, and those that are mainly or purely water (Table 11.3). Clearly, some conditions have elements of both.

When there is loss of an ECF-equivalent fluid, there is a decrease in the total ECF volume and this includes the plasma volume.

This deficit should be replaced promptly to restore perfusion to cells and vital organs. Abnormal losses of water with or without electrolytes (particularly sodium and potassium) will result not only a reduction in plasma volume but also a marked change in intracellular fluid volume and the concentrations of important ions across cell membranes. Restoration of the plasma volume always takes precedence, and should be accomplished with a 'balanced salt solution' (see below).

Restoration of the water deficit and other electrolyte deficits can then be addressed. This should be accomplished gradually so that rapid shifts of water across membranes, especially the blood/brain barrier, are avoided. It takes much longer for electrolytes to equilibrate between some compartments, and the resulting osmotic gradient can lead to fatal cerebral oedema or other complications if therapy is too hasty. Aim to correct these over 48–72 hours.

## REPLACING EXTRACELLULAR FLUID LOSS

Central to the replacement of ECF deficits (blood volume, interstitial volume) is the use of a 'balanced salt solution'. This term refers to a crystalloid solution which is isotonic (and remains so) and has constituents that are similar to the ECF, (normal saline or 0.9% sodium chloride, lactated Ringer's buffer – also known as Hartmann's solution). When a balanced salt solution is given, it will distribute itself throughout the extracellular compartment (~14 l) over several minutes. Only about a third of the volume given will remain in the vascular space. Understanding this phenomenon will prevent undertreatment of blood volume deficits when using balanced salt solutions. As reduced intravascular volume is usually accompanied by an ECF deficit, redistribution of balanced salt solution into the interstitial space is usually desirable. Normal saline contains too much chloride for physiological needs and, with over-prescription, hyperchloraemia (and acidosis) occur. Hartmann's solution does not cause this.

In a situation where the volumes required are large, maintenance water and electrolytes are often forgotten. This seldom matters in the first 24 hours or so because the volume shifts are so large and the kidney can usually sort out what it wants to keep or excrete. However, as time goes on, maintenance water needs to be thought about or the patient will become hypernatraemic and hyperosmolar.

## VOMITING, DIARRHOEA AND INTESTINAL FISTULA LOSSES

These gastrointestinal conditions cause losses of fluid which resemble ECF although typically of a lower osmolality (*i.e.* more water is lost relative to sodium). The result is blood volume depletion, dehydration, and large electrolyte losses. If water only has been taken orally to try to compensate, hyponatraemia may be present; however, if serum sodium is normal or even high, the possibility of a significant sodium deficit must not be overlooked. In some conditions (*e.g.* vomiting from complete upper small bowel obstruction, diarrhoea due to cholera) the volumes lost can be huge and rapidly life-threatening.

Potassium depletion is universal, and may be severe with marked diarrhoea. Metabolic acidosis may mask the extent of total body potassium deficit by causing potassium to move from within cells to the extracellular compartment in exchange for extracellular hydrogen ions.

Additionally, vomiting or nasogastric drainage leads to loss of hydrogen ($H^+$) and chloride ($Cl^-$) ions from the stomach. This can produce a marked metabolic alkalosis but, despite this, it is rare that $H^+$ needs to be given intravenously. Adequate chloride replacement in the form of normal saline will usually correct the deficit, as endogenously produced acid ($H^+$) will be retained by the kidney.

By using fluid balance charts and clinical assessment logically to keep total volume and key ions, particularly sodium and potassium, in balance, you can achieve success in the great majority of cases. However, there is no single formula for success and patients change continually – so re-assess!

## CASE SCENARIO 11.1

A 58-year-old, 70kg man, otherwise fit except for long-standing AF controlled with digoxin, underwent a cystectomy for bladder cancer 3 days ago. An ileal urostomy was constructed, necessitating a small bowel anastomosis. Presently, he is on HDU, is apyrexial and his chest is clear (respiratory rate 16/min), but his abdomen is rather distended. Although his urine output is rather low, he seems reasonably well perfused. The monitor shows AF at a rate of 118 bpm. It is Saturday and you are on-call – the HDU nurse has asked you to sort out his fluid balance for the weekend. Review the fluid balance chart below and prescribe his intravenous fluid. His consultant wished him to stop antibiotics after 72 h.

- WHAT FURTHER INFORMATION DO YOU REQUIRE?
- WHAT WOULD YOU PRESCRIBE AND HOW?
- ARE BLOOD TESTS NECESSARY TODAY?
- WHEN SHOULD YOU REVIEW FURTHER?

## DATA

| Intake summary | CVP line | Peripheral line (R) | Peripheral line (L) | Oral |
|---|---|---|---|---|
| (last 24 h) | Normal saline (975 ml) | Dextrose 5% (1800 ml) | Antibiotics (600 ml), PCA (125 ml) | Sips (120 ml) |

| Losses summary | Nasogastric tube | Pelvic drain | Urostomy | Bowels |
|---|---|---|---|---|
| (last 24 h) | 1450 ml | 720 ml | 640 ml | Nil, no flatus |

## CASE SCENARIO 11.1 ANSWERS

This is clearly a complex case who is not yet clinically stable. In addition to making your own clinical assessment, you should review the fluid charts from the previous day or two to look for patterns and for accumulating losses or excesses. Look at the operation note for any specific postoperative orders. Urinary anastomoses may leak for a few days – so urine appears through the drain as well as the catheter and/or urostomy. Ileus can be prolonged and nutritional support may be needed but, again, this is not pressing at 72 h postoperatively. You clearly need to review yesterday's biochemistry results (Na 138, K 3.1, urea 5.2) and repeat these today. Summate the data above and include insensible loss – about 750 ml is probably reasonable here, but revise the factors which influence this.

His needs are probably about 3500 ml – the water requirement (5% dextrose 2000 ml) will be unchanged – the excess volume should be crystalloid (1500 ml). His antibiotics will be stopped, but his PCA will continue. You will need to give at least some of the fluid via the CVP line to keep it open. He is hypokalaemic and you should aim to give 80 mmol K over the next 24 h – you may modify this when you review with the blood results later. This need is the more pressing because of his AF and digoxin therapy. If K replacement and digoxin fail to control the rate then the magnesium level should be ascertained.

It is obviously inappropriate to prescribe for the whole weekend just now. Some losses – the nasogastric loss for example – may increase or decrease and clinical and biochemical re-assessment is needed. Plan to review with your team at the end of today and again at 8 a.m. tomorrow.

## SUMMARY

- fluid and electrolyte imbalance is common and detrimental
- accurate fluid balance is achievable with a logical approach
- consider basal requirements based on patient size and age
- consider abnormal on going losses, pre-existing deficits or excesses, fluid shifts
- normal renal and cardiovascular function protect against fluid intolerance
- look at the fluid balance chart for last 24 hours. Are all fluids given or lost included? Do the volumes seem right from other available information? Check previous charts for insidious changes
- aim to correct electrolyte values – may be active or passive
- use urine electrolytes, weight and plasma osmolality when needed.

## FURTHER READING

Powell-Tuck J, Gosling P, Lobo DN *et al.*
*British Consensus Guidelines on Intravenous Fluid Therapy for Adult Surgical Patients* (*GIFTASUP*).
London: NHS National Library of Health, 2008.

# 12

## Sepsis and multiple organ failure

insults, including infection and trauma (Fig. 1). The mediators involved include nitric oxide, bradykinin, histamine, prostaglandins and cytokines, all of which have vaso-active properties. They produce a state of vasodilatation, enhanced capillary leak and eventually myocardial depression.

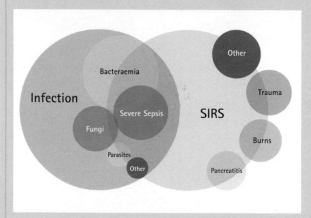

Figure 12.1 Interacting factors that result in sepsis.

The number of patients at risk of major sepsis progressively increases each year. Patients with indwelling catheters, those in ICU or HDUs, those being treated with chemotherapy or steroids, are individuals at particular risk. In addition, the ageing population and the ability to treat patients with major chronic illness increases the complexity of management of patients with sepsis. In the US at present, septic shock is estimated to account for about 100,000 deaths annually and the mortality has changed little in the past 30 years; the mortality of surgical patients with major sepsis/septic shock continues at the level of about 50%.

It is important to recognise that the signs and symptoms associated with sepsis are caused by the release of endogenous mediators. This mediator release may be precipitated by a variety if

Cytokines involved include interleukin-1 (endogenous pyrogen), tumour necrosis factor and interleukin-6. Released from the patient's own white blood cells, these contribute to the patient's pyrexia and hypermetabolic state. While production of mediators is needed to combat infection, an excessive or prolonged activation of such cellular and humoral mediator pathways is thought to contribute to the development of multiple organ failure (MOF) in patients with major sepsis.

A balance exists between inadequate and excessive responses to infection. Inter-individual variation in the pattern of mediator release and of end-organ responsiveness plays a significant role in determining the initial physiological response to major sepsis and this may be a determinant of outcome. Other important prognostic features include the severity of the initial 'trigger event', the timeliness and adequacy of treatment of the underlying condition and the patient's general state of health.

## DEFINITIONS

The systemic inflammatory response syndrome (SIRS) and sepsis is a spectrum of illness ranging from mild systemic disturbance (typically seen in the early postoperative patient) to life-threatening multiple organ failure. A consensus conference (Barcelona, 2001) agreed the now accepted definitions outlined in Table 12.1. All involve a systemic derangement which distinguishes them from localised infection.

As described above, many surgical patients have evidence of SIRS, and the vast majority

---

### TABLE 12.1

#### CONSENSUS CONFERENCE DEFINITIONS IN SEPSIS

**Systemic inflammatory response syndrome**
**(SIRS, also known as symptoms and signs of infection or SSI)**
Two or more of:
- pyrexia (> 38˚C) or hypothermia (< 36˚C)
- tachycardia (> 90 bpm in absence of ß-blocker)
- tachypnoea (> 20 breaths per minute or a requirement for mechanical ventilation)
- white cell count > 12 or < 4
- acutely altered mental state
- blood glucose of > 6.6 in the absence of diabetes

Sepsis = SIRS + documented source of infection

**Severe sepsis (confirmed infection) or sepsis syndrome (no confirmed infection)**
SIRS + altered organ perfusion or evidence of dysfunction of one or more organs. Almost any organ or system can be involved, including:
- CVS (lactate > 1.2 mmol/1 or SVR < 800 dyne/s/cm$^3$)
- respiratory (PaO$_2$/FiO$_2$ < 30 or PaO$_2$ < 9.3 kPa)
- renal (urine output < 120 ml over 4 h)
- CNS (GCS < 15 in absence of sedation/neurological lesion).

It is important to note that the identification of organ dysfunction is initially a clinical diagnosis. You should think about organ dysfunction/failure in any critically ill surgical patient who looks breathless, has poor perfusion, confusion, poor urine output or abnormal coagulation.

**Septic shock**
Refractory hypotension in addition to the above, in the presence of invasive infection

---

will recover uneventfully with good surgical care. However, the presence of such signs, particularly when persistent, serves as a warning of the potential for deterioration in the absence of prompt treatment. SIRS may result from an infective process or other conditions, including pancreatitis, ischaemia, multiple trauma or haemorrhagic shock.

When such a response is due to an identified infective process, it is known as sepsis; when it is associated with organ dysfunction, hypoperfusion or hypotension, it is termed severe sepsis (infective cause) or sepsis syndrome (no identified infection).

The septic picture can be caused by surgical and non-surgical factors and, as indicated above, can occur with confirmed infection or in its absence. Although specific criteria for organ dysfunction exist, you should be actively looking for clinical evidence of organ derangement (*e.g.* dyspnoea, hypoxia, oliguria, jaundice, thromobocytopenia) in all susceptible patients.

The essential points of management of the patient with sepsis include:
- early recognition
- immediate resuscitation
- localisation of sepsis
- early and appropriate administration of antibiotics
- appropriate management of the primary source of sepsis including the use of surgical or radiological drainage
- on going re-assessment to ensure the patient continues to improve.

Failure to accomplish any of these promptly will markedly worsen the prognosis.

Table 12.2 shows some causes which you will encounter. The classification might help you

## TABLE 12.2

### POTENTIAL CAUSES OF SIRS

|  | Infective | Non-infective |
|---|---|---|
| Non-surgical | Pulmonary<br>Urinary and catheter-related<br>Intravenous lines, especially CVP<br>Soft tissue infection | Acute pancreatitis<br>Re-perfusion injury |
| Surgical | Anastomotic leak<br>Biliary especially if obstructed<br>Urinary with obstruction<br>Collection/abscess<br>Infected prosthesis (hip, aortic graft, heart valve, neurosurgical shunt)<br>Necrotic tissue | Ischaemic gut<br>Ruptured aorta<br>Major haemorrhage<br>Trauma |

remember them but a number of the causes could appear in different boxes depending on the stage (*e.g.* ischaemic gut). Surgical ones often require a surgical solution but all causes occur in surgical patients.

## PATIENT ASSESSMENT AND MANAGEMENT

### IMMEDIATE CARE

Remember the ABCs: patients with major sepsis may have a tachypnoea and have cardiovascular changes. The presence of these changes demands high-flow oxygen via a facemask and establishment of intravenous access with volume expansion by appropriate fluid bolus at a minimum.

### FULL PATIENT ASSESSMENT

*Chart review*

Vital signs should be reviewed carefully: tachypnoea, tachycardia, hypo- or hyperthermia are all consistent with sepsis. A CVP between 5–10 cmH$_2$O and a urine output greater than 30 ml/h are reasonable guides to the adequacy of initial fluid resuscitation. If hypotension/inadequate perfusion persists despite adequate fluid replacement and CVP monitoring, then inotropic support should be considered, which will require input from colleagues experienced in critical care and involve additional monitoring.

*History and systematic examination*

An assessment of the patient's presenting complaint may help to establish the likely source of sepsis:

- breathlessness and a productive cough may indicate a pulmonary source
- abdominal pain or bowel symptoms may point to an abdominal problem. An abdominal or pelvic abscess may cause diarrhoea or an ileus: anastomotic leaks are common and can be subtle
- frequency, dysuria or haematuria are common in urinary sepsis, which can often implicate the urinary tract. Beware the combination of obstruction with infection (usually due to a stone), as sepsis may be severe and permanent renal damage can occur rapidly
- headache and neck stiffness may point to a source in the central nervous system. Remember, however, that confusion is common in the unwell septic patient and does not necessarily indicate a source in the CNS.

The systemic review should also evaluate chronic health problems and current medication which may suggest a susceptibility to sepsis (*e.g.* use of steroids) or may indicate the need for more intensive monitoring (*e.g.* recent myocardial infarction).

The history and examination may be very useful in helping to indicate the source of the problem. Common things occur frequently: chest infection, anastomotic leak, central line infection are often implicated in the recovering surgical patient. Timing of events can also help: the chest is a common early cause of postoperative fever or sepsis from day 1 onwards while anastomotic leak, as mentioned previously, usually occurs from day 4 and central line infection becomes more frequent in lines more than 48 hours old.

## CASE SCENARIO 12.1

As the surgical trainee on the HDU 8 a.m. ward round, you review a 73-year-old woman with mild COAD who had a left hemicolectomy with primary anastomosis for colonic carcinoma 6 days ago. You are told that the white blood cell count was 16.3 yesterday, increased from 8.5 the day before.

### WHAT WOULD YOU DO?

Systematic assessment shows that her ABCs are stable. The charts show an increased heart rate (was 70 bpm, now 95 bpm), a temporary pyrexia of 38°C over night and decreased urine output (only 25 ml/h for the last 3 h). The patient has no specific complaints but has been generally slow to recover. The CVP line is still *in situ*, as is the epidural and the urinary catheter. Examination of her chest is unchanged, and shows a few basal crackles, but stable gas exchange and she is able to expectorate adequately without pain. Her abdomen is slightly distended, and flatus has been passed but no faeces. There is no evidence of a DVT. Macroscopically and on 'dipstick', her urine is clear.

### WHAT WOULD YOU DO NOW?

Now is the time to decide and plan! The patient is not quite right but has no definite signs. There are a number of potential sources of sepsis (chest, CVP line, urine, urinary catheter, abdomen, anastomosis). Peripheral blood cultures and cultures through the central venous line should be sent, as should urine and sputum cultures. A chest X-ray should be ordered if there is not a recent one, a fluid challenge started and the physiotherapist called.

When reviewing such a case, the operation performed (which includes a primary colonic anastomosis), the stage of recovery and the fact that her gut has still not started working again should make you consider an anastomotic leak. You discuss the case with your consultant and arrange a contrast-enhanced CT scan. A small, localised leak is suspected. Your consultant thinks that the patient may settle, and takes a conservative approach to further management. Antibiotics are prescribed and the patient is fasted.

### ON REVIEW

Overall, the patient appears to remain unchanged throughout the next 24 h. There is one further flicker of pyrexia (37.8°C). The heart rate remains at 95–100 bpm. The next morning, her abdomen is still distended and her ileus persists. The urea has climbed to 10.4 and patient had a run of fast AF at 5 a.m. despite a CVP of +9 and normal saturations. 12-lead ECG and cardiac enzymes were normal but Mg level was low. This has been corrected.

Your consultant joins you and together you decide that the failure to respond (abdomen, heart rate) and the recent cardiac and renal effects are more than enough to require surgery to deal with the leak. After appropriate resuscitation, she is taken to theatre where the anastomosis is taken down and the ends exteriorised. The patient returns to HDU and makes an uncomplicated further recovery.

> **LEARNING POINTS**
>
> The causes of postoperative pyrexia and of sepsis in surgical patients are not the same:
> - anastomotic leaks are not uncommon
>   they may present with a variety of features, often between day 4 and day 8
> - symptoms range from the catastrophic collapse into MOF to subtle derangements of vital signs or biochemical parameters, or 'failure to progress'
> - gut function is usually delayed or absent (but not always!)
> - surgical or radiological intervention is often required
> - organ dysfunction requires prompt action
> - the intervention required depends on the site and the previous operation but leaking small bowel and colonic anastomoses are usually best exteriorised as stomas.

*Available results*

Review available results and arrange new investigations.

The white blood cell count may be abnormally high (> 10 x 10$^9$/l) or low (< 2 x 10$^9$/l) in major sepsis. A coagulation screen should be checked, particularly if surgery is contemplated: thrombocytopenia and coagulopathies are common and should be corrected before surgery.

The urea and electrolytes should be reviewed with particular attention to renal function: acute renal failure is a frequent complication of severe sepsis and is often preventable in the early stages by adequate fluid resuscitation.

Liver function tests may be abnormal, particularly when the biliary tree is the primary source of sepsis or as part of a multi-organ failure syndrome (MOFS).

An ECG should be checked for evidence of ischaemia or arrhythmia.

ABGs should be taken and may show hypoxaemia, with or without a metabolic acidosis.

Aerobic and anaerobic blood cultures are obligatory but will only be positive in about 20% of cases. A higher positive culture rate can be achieved if the primary source of sepsis can be cultured (*e.g.* pus from an abscess, urine from an infected system). Sputum, urine, drain fluid and pus from wounds should be sent for culture and sensitivity. Cultures should also be taken through in-dwelling central venous catheters. Fungal infection should be considered, particularly when the diagnosis is proving elusive or there have been multiple previous courses of antibiotics. Empirical treatment with antibiotics can be started on an 'educated guess' basis (with advice from the microbiologists locally). These can be changed when results of culture and antibiotic sensitivity become available.

Further evaluation of possible sites of sepsis include the use of ultrasound, CT scanning and laparotomy. Remember the adage, 'pus somewhere, pus nowhere, pus under the diaphragm'. Patients who are immunocompromised (*e.g.* transplant patients) may develop opportunistic infections which may require very specific investigation (*e.g.* broncho-alveolar lavage or transbronchial biopsy for those with pneumonia).

## DAILY MANAGEMENT PLAN: THE STABLE PATIENT

A daily management plan is needed for all patients, no matter how stable they appear to be. This ensures that all members of the multidisciplinary team know what is going to happen. A list of clear, positive decisions listed in the patient record provides a plan for genuine progress. The aim is to ensure progress through attention to detail and gives the patient the best chance of avoiding further deterioration. Features to consider include the following.

*Fluids*
It is important to hydrate all patients adequately to allow good tissue perfusion. Crystalloids are usually appropriate fluid replacement: colloids may remain in the circulation longer but, when they escape to the tissues, may worsen oedema. Patients with sepsis syndrome may require up to 10–12 l of fluid in the first 24 hours of resuscitation.

## CASE SCENARIO 12.2

A 61-year-old, previously fit, woman was admitted to the ward 4 days ago with acute sigmoid diverticulitis. Initial signs included minimal tenderness in the left iliac fossa. Treatment was started with a second generation cephalsosporin and metronidazole. Fever and leukocytosis settled within 48 h. She has suddenly become acutely unwell, with recurrent tenderness in the left iliac fossa, pyrexia of 39.2°C, tachycardia and hypotension.

**WHAT WOULD YOU DO AT THIS STAGE? WHAT IS YOUR DIFFERENTIAL DIAGNOSIS?**
It is clear that the patient has deteriorated markedly despite initial treatment for her presumed diagnosis: a change of treatment is needed. Following resuscitation (including blood cultures and biochemical tests) and after discussion with her consultant, an experienced surgical trainee takes the patient to theatre for an emergency sigmoid colectomy. There is a 7 cm pelvic abscess beside the inflamed sigmoid colon, which is drained and a sample of pus sent for urgent microbiological examination and culture. A Hartmann's procedure (sigmoid colectomy with colostomy and closure of the rectal stump) is carried out and the patient returned to HDU in stable condition. Peri-operative antibiotics were given as previously and prescribed for a further 5 days.

### LEARNING POINTS

- anticipate – from the initial diagnosis and your knowledge of common complications
- resuscitate adequately – monitor and get help as necessary
- cultures – blood and source
- antibiotics – best guess then selective and in short courses
- definitive surgical treatment is essential.

Care should be taken to avoid fluid overload, and such large volume fluid resuscitation is likely to require guidance by using additional monitoring (*e.g.* CVP or cardiac output monitoring).

*Oxygen*
It is essential that the patient does not become hypoxaemic: oxygen should be administered as required to correct hypoxaemia. If facemask oxygen is inadequate, consideration should be given to additional respiratory support, which will usually require help from ICU colleagues.

*Nutrition*
It is essential to ensure adequate metabolic and nutritional support of the patient in order to optimise the patient's endogenous immune function. This can be by the enteral or parenteral route.

*Antibiotics*
Antibiotics must be given as early as possible. Empirical treatment on a 'best-guess' basis should be started with microbiological advice. It is important to review the microbiology after 48 hours when cultures are available and sensitivities obtained; discussing cases with the microbiologist can be very helpful and is to be recommended. It has been shown clearly that the mortality of patients is significantly lower when appropriate antibiotics are prescribed early in the course of the patient's illness. It is also important to appreciate that fungi and atypical organisms can contribute to the sepsis syndrome and to take cultures and prescribe appropriately. Prolonged 'prophylaxis' is not recommended, as 'super-infection' by fungi and antibiotic-resistant organisms is encouraged. Finally, remember that enteric streptococci account for 10–20% of severe infections related to the abdomen and that they are not sensitive to all common prophylactic antibiotics.

*Additional considerations*
Instructions for physiotherapy, DVT prophylaxis and, in a patient with ongoing abdominal sepsis, drain management should also be included in the daily management plan.

## DIAGNOSING CAUSE OF DETERIORATION: THE UNSTABLE PATIENT
In a patient with new or ongoing sepsis, deterioration may be elicited by pyrexia, clotting disturbances, a metabolic acidosis and/or organ dysfunction. Alternatively, the patient may simply fail to progress. The presence of such a pattern demands careful clinical review of symptoms and signs, repeat microbiology, review of antibiotic sensitivities and may require further radiological evaluation with either percutaneous or operative drainage of localised sepsis. Failure to diagnose significant sepsis will prove fatal.

*Definitive treatment*
Definitive treatment is the single most important factor in securing survival. Localised collections of pus generally need either operative or percutaneous drainage and dead tissue should be excised.

Severe pulmonary sepsis requires adequate antibiotics and chest physiotherapy. It may also require repeat bronchoscopy and toilet of the bronchial tree, and additional respiratory support (NIV, IPPV).

In spreading soft tissue infection, it is important to establish adequate drainage and vital to excise necrotic or devitalised tissue as well as giving antibiotics. Repeated examination under anaesthesia with further debridement is usually needed.

Abdominal sepsis, if localised, may be treated initially with antibiotics or percutaneous drainage, but generally the primary source of sepsis must be removed. Copious intra-operative peritoneal lavage is important and you should be alert to the development of recurrent sepsis during subsequent assessments of the patient.

A planned, second-look laparotomy may be useful, particularly in patients with equivocal bowel perfusion during previous procedures.

Obstruction of the biliary or urinary system must be relieved. An infected prosthesis will usually need to be removed (*e.g.* peripheral or central venous cannulae, urinary catheters, prosthetic metalwork). Sometimes, such decisions are difficult and will require discussion between different medical teams. Vigilance around the possibility of catheter-associated sepsis, particularly in patients in the HDU or ICU, is essential.

MRSA infection is becoming more common in all patients. It is important to distinguish between patients who are colonised carriers and those with MRSA sepsis. Whereas MRSA colonisation does not present major problems in most patients, it may do in those patients with prostheses (aortic valves, aortic grafts, hip replacements) where it is associated with a very high mortality. Often, the only treatment is removal of the prosthesis and long-term antibiotics. Microbiological help is essential.

## PREVENT – DIAGNOSE – ACT
### THE SURVIVING SEPSIS CAMPAIGN
The Surviving Sepsis Campaign (SSC), a collaborative initiative developed by 11 international societies, was launched in 2002.

The aim of the SSC is to reduce mortality from severe sepsis. Initial guidelines were announced in 2004, and updated in early 2008 to respond to latest evidence.

The SSC includes two recommended management packages or 'care bundles' – the Resuscitation Care Bundle and the Management Care Bundle.

*The SSC Resuscitation Care Bundle*
The Resuscitation Care Bundle aims to optimise the care of patients with sepsis during the first 6 hours from onset of symptoms. It starts with the 'Sepsis Six' – six tasks easily performed by non-specialist staff, which provide the crucial first steps in delivering the care bundle:

### THE SEPSIS SIX
Give high-flow oxygen
Take blood cultures
Give intravenous antibiotics
Start intravenous fluid resuscitation
Check haemoglobin and lactate levels
Measure accurate hourly urine output

Following the 'Sepsis Six', the SSC recommends that patients with persistent hypotension or increased lactate should be managed with early goal directed therapy (EGDT). EGDT will require input from your critical care colleagues or other senior doctors, but the principles used are important to recognise and are outlined below.

*SSC Management Care Bundle*
Following initial resuscitation, the SSC has recommendations for the next 24 hours of

## SURVIVING SEPSIS CAMPAIGN SEPSIS RESUSCITATION CARE BUNDLE

- Measure serum lactate
- Get blood cultures before giving antibiotics
- From the time of presentation, give broad spectrum antibiotics:
  - within 3 h for emergency department admissions
  - within 1 h for non-emergency department, ICU admissions
- In the event of hypotension or lactate > 4 mmol/l:
  - deliver an initial minimum of 20 ml/kg of crystalloid (or colloid equivalent)
  - apply vasopressors for hypotension not responding to initial fluid resuscitation to maintain mean arterial pressure of 65 mmHg
- In the event of persistent hypotension despite fluid resuscitation (septic shock) or lactate > 4 mmol/l:
  - achieve CVP of 8 mmHg
  - achieve central venous oxygen saturation of > 70%
- These tasks should begin immediately and must be done within 6 h for patients with severe sepsis or septic shock.

treatment. The Management Care Bundle includes specialist critical care treatment and strategies proven to improve patient outcome. Although outside the remit of the CCrISP course, these therapies include the use of activated protein C when indicated, 'tight' glycaemic control and limitation of ventilatory pressures when using positive pressure ventilation.

## MANAGEMENT OF MULTIPLE ORGAN FAILURE

Due to the severity of the initial insult or when there is a persistence of an activated systemic inflammatory response, a patient may develop dysfunction or failure of one or more organ systems (cardiovascular, pulmonary, renal, gut, liver, haematological, CNS). When 3 or more systems have failed, the ensuing mortality approaches 80–100%. Once one organ system has failed, others typically follow – like a collapsing pack of cards (see case scenario). It is important to appreciate the phenomenon of multi-organ failure and to support each organ system to avoid further adverse events (*e.g.* ventilation, haemofiltration/ haemodialysis, inotropic support, nutritional support, use of blood products).

Respiratory failure may be the result of infection (often added to pre-existing chronic airway disease) or adult respiratory distress syndrome (ARDS). ARDS is a diffuse, inflammatory process, usually involving both lungs, and is often seen as part of a sepsis syndrome associated with any underlying cause. The lungs become 'waterlogged' due to extravasation of inflammatory fluid and cells. Patients may develop ARDS quickly, deteriorating rapidly over a few hours. Pulmonary signs are often minimal or non-specific: patients are breathless, becoming progressively tachypnoeic and hypoxic. A chest X-ray will show bilateral infiltrates but this may lag behind the clinical picture. Respiratory support is almost always needed (usually IPPV) and expert ICU help should be obtained at an early stage. Suspicion is the key to diagnosing ARDS.

Cardiovascular failure in MOF results from 3 main factors: (i) loss of peripheral vascular tone (vasodilatation); (ii) loss of circulating volume

## CASE SCENARIO 12.3

When on call, you are asked to review the patient discussed above (Case Scenario 12.2) 72 h following surgery. She had improved for 48 h and was returned to the ward, but is now breathless and pyrexial again (38.3°C), having been apyrexial since 4 h after surgery. Blood pressure is normal but she is tachycardic (115 bpm), tachypnoeic (28/min) and poorly perfused. Urine output has fallen off over the last 4 h to 12 ml in the last hour. The chest seems clear. Her abdomen is distended and quiet. The stoma has not worked properly yet. The pelvic drain has produced 40 ml serous fluid today only. You give high flow oxygen (12 l/min) and start a fluid challenge of 500 ml saline stat.

The foundation year doctor had checked bloods and a chest X-ray. Apart from a leukocytosis (17,000), results are unremarkable. There are no diagnostic features on the chest X-ray. There are no signs of DVT and prescribed DVT prophylaxis (s.c. heparin and TED stockings) were in place. You perform a cautious rectal examination but find no obvious abnormality. Blood gases are now checked and show $PaO_2$ (on $FiO_2$ of 0.6) 11.4 kPa, pH 7.29, BE −7.2. You move the patient to HDU. When the results come back, you decide that the patient has been acidotic and hypoxic and that you have barely corrected the hypoxia with the facemask oxygen. After 1000 ml of saline, there is a little improvement in perfusion, but no change in heart rate and urine output is only 15 ml in the hour since you were called.

### WHAT WOULD YOU DO NOW? WHAT IS YOUR DIFFERENTIAL DIAGNOSIS?

The patient remains breathless and you have neither a diagnosis nor any further intervention of obvious help at your disposal. You request an urgent review by ICU and, as the patient still seems underperfused, give a further fluid challenge, while the foundation year doctor checks an ECG (normal).

The ICU team arrive and assess the patient They share your concern and think ventilation will be needed – transfer is arranged. You inform your consultant, who asks to be kept informed. During transfer, the patient becomes more breathless and is intubated shortly after arriving in ICU. The positive pressure ventilation reduces cardiac filling and, despite further fluid loading, inotropes are required to support the cardiovascular system. Urine output tails off. A chest X-ray shows some diffuse bilateral shadowing suggestive of ARDS. You update your consultant who comes to examine the patient. No cause for deterioration has yet been found.

Given the previous operation and the leukocytosis, recurrent abdominal sepsis is suspected. The patient is too unstable for CT, so repeat laparotomy is arranged and carried out by the consultant. The bowel is intact but two abscesses are found between loops of small intestine and a left subphrenic abscess is identified: these are drained and lavaged. More pus is sent for culture.

The patient returns to ICU for full cardiac, respiratory and renal support. The culture result from the pus taken at the first operation has grown a coliform resistant to prescribed antibiotics but sensitive to netilmicin. Treatment is changed accordingly and a 7-day course started. The patient slowly begins to improve over the succeeding 72 hours.

**LEARNING POINTS**

Remember the SSC: Prevent, Diagnose, Act

- sepsis can progress rapidly – an escalating degree of support, often out of working hours, may be required. Your role is to recognise and treat the many patients with 'minor' sepsis who respond adequately on the ward, but also to recognise the patient who is not responding and who needs ICU help
- a diagnosis which accounts adequately for any septic deterioration is essential – this allows definitive treatment ('source control')
- early cultures can help target later treatment – the right antibiotic is important.

due to leaky capillaries (hypovolaemia); and (iii) myocardial depression (pump failure). Arrhythmias can exert a further effect. Close monitoring of cardiovascular status is essential to guide treatment adequately. Fluid resuscitation may prove successful, although inotropic and vasopressor support is often required. Many intensivists use noradrenaline to increase peripheral vascular tone, often in conjunction with other agents to increase cardiac contractility.

Renal failure which is common in MOF is often established during the early stages of the condition before hypovolaemia is corrected. Circulating nephrotoxins may compound this. Although renal function usually improves when the patient recovers, renal replacement therapy may be required during the period of MOF and for some time afterwards. Failure of other systems occurs (gut, brain, clotting system) may be due to direct effects of the pathology or to systemic inflammation and hypoxia. For there to be any prospect of recovery, the underlying cause or source of sepsis must be treated.

Nosocomial (hospital acquired) infection is common in patients treated in ICU and may compound MOF. The decision to give antibiotics for a positive culture (*e.g.* of *Pseudomonas* spp.) should be carefully balanced by the presence of a host response to such bacteria, the site of the potential infection and the need to avoid superinfection or antibiotic resistance. Such issues should be discussed with the microbiologist.

The recognition of the role of endogenous mediators in sepsis syndrome and the advent of biotechnology resulted in several, large, multicentre, randomised trials using monoclonal antibodies or antagonists to various sepsis mediators including activated protein C, endotoxin, tumour necrosis factor and interleukin-1. However, it remains clear that these treatments are unlikely ever to replace the established basic principles of management, although time will tell whether a substantial adjuvant role can be identified.

## CASE SCENARIO 12.4

The patient again deteriorates overnight, needing increased vasopressors, inotropic support and oxygen, highly suggestive of sepsis. A full infection screen has been taken by the time you arrive and the central lines have been changed by your ICU colleagues. There are no clinical features to suggest recurrent intra-abdominal sepsis: an abdominal CT confirms there is no new intra-abdominal collection. The patient has had several recent courses of antibiotics and there is no clear 'best-guess' antibiotic to use.

### WHAT IS YOUR DIFFERENTIAL DIAGNOSIS?

6 hours later, the patient is no better and a joint discussion is held between surgeons, ICU staff and the microbiologist. No cultures are available but fungi were seen on samples from the urinary catheter and one of the removed central lines. It is decided to start treatment with amphotericin and fluconazole for presumed fungal sepsis.

After a 4-week course and several other complications, the patient is discharged to the ward.

### LEARNING POINTS

- Surgical patients on ICU with sepsis and MOF run a roller-coaster course, often with a range of complications – some surgical and some medical. An active surgical input to care helps manage these effectively.
- Multiple courses of antibiotics, gastrointestinal perforation, critical illness and multiple monitoring lines are all risk factors for fungal sepsis – many of these factors pertain in a majority of surgical patients.
- Fungal sepsis may present with obscure signs – a failure to progress. Identification of fungi within the blood, abdomen or urine (or at any 2 other sites) would prompt many intensivists to discuss antifungal therapy with their microbiologist and surgeon.

Established septic shock or MOF is thus really only treatable by prevention through attention to detail.

Pre-operatively, the general health of the patient should be optimised (co-existing diseases, nutrition) and any focus of sepsis should be treated. Peri-operatively, prophylactic antibiotics should be given and surgery executed in a rapid, clean and haemostatic manner in order to prevent complications. Operations should be performed electively whenever possible.

Postoperatively, assess clinically and monitor closely to detect problems at an early stage and deal with these quickly and comprehensively. Be alert to 'occult' hypoxia and hypovolaemia. Use prophylactic measures such as chest physiotherapy and resume oral intake/enteral feeding at the earliest opportunity. Remove lines and tubes as soon as possible, and employ short courses of targeted antibiotics. In the event of a septic complication, adequate resuscitation and early definitive treatment should reduce the chance of full-blown sepsis developing.

## SUMMARY

- sepsis is a mediator disease
- prevention is better than cure
- clinical signs may be obvious, but are often covert
- treatment is much easier at an early stage
- the principles of management are:
  (i) rapid resuscitation to restore oxygenation and perfusion;
  (ii) continued optimal organ support;
  (iii) diagnosis and eradication of the source of sepsis and any pus;
  (iv) judicious and appropriate antibiotic treatment after cultures; and
  (v) re-assessment to ensure continued progress
- the SSC guidelines, particularly the 'Sepsis Six', are a useful starting point in the management of the patient with severe sepsis.

# 13

## Nutrition in the surgical patient

Malnutrition occurs when there is a deficiency of energy, proteins, vitamins and minerals causing effects on body function and/or clinical outcomes. It can occur in surgical patients either as a cause or as result of the surgical condition.

Malnutrition is a common finding in surgical patients: as many as 50% of patients on general surgical wards are reported to have evidence of protein-energy malnutrition (PEM). Although, in many cases, these effects may be due to the nature of the disease process itself rather than malnutrition, it is important to ensure that, wherever possible, inadequate nutritional intake does not add to the likelihood of a poor outcome in critically ill and postoperative patients.

# INDICATIONS FOR NUTRITIONAL SUPPORT

Nutritional support should be considered for all malnourished patients. Malnourished patients are defined by NICE as those with:

- a BMI of less than 18.5 kg/m$^2$
- an unintentional weight loss greater than 10% within the last 3–6 months
- a BMI less than 20 kg/m$^2$ and unintentional weight loss greater than 5% within the last 3–6 months.

Surgical patients at risk of malnutrition should also be considered for nutritional support if they have:

- not had, or are not likely to have, significant oral intake for more than 5 days, or
- a poor absorptive capacity, high nutrient losses or increased nutritional needs due to increased catabolic rate.

In many critically ill patients (notably those with SIRS and sepsis), the underlying problem relates to impaired utilisation of fuel substrates, rather than an absolute deficiency, and no amount of externally-added nutrients will reverse the process which is consuming the body's reserves. Efforts must, therefore, be directed to identifying and treating the underlying cause, including any source of infection or necrotic tissue.

Nutritional support should be considered for every surgical patient unable to resume adequate dietary intake for more than 3–5 days and in every critically ill patient, although its benefit may not be realised until the underlying disease process settles. If the gastrointestinal tract is working and access to it can be safely obtained, enteral feeding should be initiated. It is cheaper, safer, and has physiological advantages over alternative methods of support. The barrier function of the small intestine deteriorates if luminal nutrients are not provided. This may increase the ability of bacteria and endotoxins to cross the intestinal wall, and possibly contribute to the development of multiple organ failure. The villous height, which determines the mass and surface area of the small bowel, also decreases rapidly, increasing the risk of diarrhoea on resumption of feeding. This, in turn, may delay introduction of oral feeding, compounding the situation. Furthermore, liver dysfunction, hyperglycaemia and septic complications, especially chest infections, are significantly less common with enteral feeding compared to parenteral nutrition.

Nutritional support must be an integral part of good surgical and critical care support. Consideration must be given to the duration of support required. In patients with simple starvation, considered for elective surgical intervention, nutritional support needs to be given for a minimum of 2 weeks pre-operatively before any significant benefit can be anticipated.

## CALCULATING NUTRITIONAL REQUIREMENTS

Nutrition support should include consideration of:
- energy, protein, fluid, electrolyte, mineral, micronutrient and fibre requirements
- any underlying condition (e.g. pyrexia)
- the likely duration of need for nutritional support.

Energy requirements can be satisfied in the form of fats, glucose or protein, which provide: fats, 9.3 kcal/g; glucose, 4.1 kcal/g; and protein, 4.1 kcal/g. There are several disadvantages in using glucose as the major energy source, so at least 50% is provided in the form of fat. Critically ill patients are often glucose intolerant and excess undergoes

hepatic conversion to lipid causing fatty liver and derangement of liver function tests. Also, carbohydrates have a higher respiratory quotient than fat and protein, producing a greater proportion of $CO_2$ to $O_2$ consumed, which can increase ventilatory requirements and contribute to respiratory dysfunction.

The 'essential' amino acids (e.g. leucine, methionine) and minerals (zinc, magnesium, etc.), which cannot be synthesized in the body, must be incorporated into nutritional support.

A basic nutritional prescription is included in Table 13.1.

### TABLE 13.1

A BASIC NUTRITIONAL PRESCRIPTION
- 30 kcal/kg/day total energy
- 0.8–1.5 g protein/kg/day (equivalent to 0.15–0.3 g nitrogen/kg/day)
- 30–35 ml/kg fluid
- essential amino acids, adequate electrolytes,
- essential minerals and micronutrients

Clearly, critically ill patients will require more nitrogen in the form of protein, more energy and probably more fluid. Nutritional support must, therefore, be calculated on an individual basis. People who have been ill or malnourished for some time and who require additional feeding, should initially not be given their full energy requirements as they are at risk for developing 'refeeding syndrome' (see below). It is safe to start feeding at 50% of estimated protein and calorie requirements and build up to full requirements over a 24–48 hour period. This only applies to the energy component of the prescription.

# ROUTES OF ENTERAL FEEDING

## SUPPLEMENTARY ENTERAL FEEDING

Supplementation of the diet with 'sip feeds' may be very useful when patients have a poor appetite but are able to drink. Sip feeds are therefore useful in people who can swallow safely but are malnourished or at risk of malnutrition. Current sip feeds typically provide 200 kcal and 2 g of nitrogen per 200 ml and are available in a variety of flavours. They may be useful in enabling patients to make the transition back to a full diet and there is some evidence to suggest that they may reduce hospital stay and increase the speed of postoperative recovery. However, they are often used to replace, rather than supplement, food intake and, despite manufacturers' best efforts, many patients still find them unpalatable. Offering sip feeds chilled and in a variety of flavours can help, along with encouraging nursing staff to offer normal oral nutrition at mealtimes in addition to supplements. Multivitamin and mineral supplements can be used to ensure there are sufficient micronutrients in the diet (Table 13.2).

---

### TABLE 13.2

#### BASIC RULES FOR ENTERAL NUTRITION

**Enteral nutritional support should be considered when:**

- spontaneous oral intake is inadequate
- the proximal small intestine is intact and functional
- stimulation of secretory function does not clearly worsen the condition being treated (*e.g.* proximal small bowel fistula).

**Contra-indications (relative and absolute) include:**

- complete small bowel obstruction
- inadequately treated shock states (may be associated with a risk of intestinal ischaemia)
- severe diarrhoea (low rate of feeding may be continued as it may improve absorptive surface)
- proximal small intestinal fistulae
- severe pancreatitis (unless fed distal to pancreas).

---

## NASOGASTRIC FEEDING

Feeding through a nasogastric tube is the easiest means of enteral feeding, but is reliant on the adequacy of gastric emptying, which is one of the last aspects of gut function to recover after an operation or major insult. High gastric residuals and gastric distension predispose to vomiting or regurgitation and aspiration. Any impairment of consciousness greatly increases this risk. Keeping the patient at least 15° head up may reduce this risk significantly.

Judging when gastric emptying is adequate can be difficult. In the fed state, the stomach can produce up to 2500 ml of secretions (in addition to receiving 1500 ml of saliva). The normal gastric residual volume is between 50–100 ml, which represents the equilibrium between secretion, and emptying plus absorption. Continuous passive drainage or suction through a conventional wide-bore nasogastric tube may lead to a large cumulative total over 24 hours even in the face of normal gastric emptying, because the gastric residual is replaced as quickly as it is removed. Pinning the bag up at shoulder height or spigotting the tube and aspirating at 2-, 4- or 6-hourly intervals will give a better indication of whether the stomach is emptying adequately. Most stresses and illnesses, plus some drugs, increase gastric residual volume, but may not necessarily lead to a degree of impaired emptying that would prevent feeding. Feeding can be commenced through a standard, large-bore nasogastric drainage tube, but a fine-bore tube is better tolerated once the need for drainage has passed. Aspiration of gastric fluid through a fine-bore tube is much more difficult, and confirmation of tube position is mandatory because of the devastating consequences of instilling feeding solution into the lung (as highlighted by the National Patient Safety Agency). Tube position must be confirmed either by checking the pH of gastric contents aspirated from a large-bore tube, or radiographic confirmation.

## NASOJEJUNAL OR NASODUODENAL FEEDING

Where gastric emptying remains a problem or direct intragastric feeding is undesirable, such as in severe pancreatitis, a weighted tube should be used and guided into the proximal small intestine. If undergoing surgery, this can be placed intra-operatively, but other options include the use of fluoroscopy to advance the tube beyond the pylorus, endoscopic placement or the use of specially designed tubes that are propelled distally by peristalsis. Prokinetic drugs such as erythromycin and metoclopramide that promote gastric motility may also be given to encourage forward movement of the tube beyond the pylorus.

## TUBE ENTEROSTOMY

Where patients are undergoing laparotomy, consideration should be given to the insertion of a tube enterostomy as a planned part of the procedure. For example, tube jejunostomy should be considered in patients undergoing oesophagectomy, total gastrectomy or pancreaticoduodenectomy or a laparotomy for abdominal trauma. For other patients, insertion of feeding tubes should be considered when it is clear that enteral nutritional support is indicated and is going to be required for more than 6 weeks. Tube gastrostomy can be fashioned using either the Stamm (pure string suture) or Witzel (seromuscular tunnel) techniques. Tube jejunostomy can also be accomplished using a catheter introduced over a fine needle, passed submucosally before entering the bowel. In all cases, the bowel should be sutured to the abdominal wall deep to the site at which the catheter passes through. Minimal access techniques can also be used. Percutaneous endoscopic gastrostomy (PEG) and transgastric jejunostomy are appropriate in the management of patients in whom laparotomy is not indicated but who need enteral nutritional support for a prolonged period.

## TABLE 13.3

### COMPLICATIONS OF PEG FEEDING

| Condition | Action | Incidence |
|---|---|---|
| Infection at PEG site | Keep clean and dry. If pain ± pus, swab and treat with antibiotics | 4% |
| Mechanical problems<br>– Blockage<br>– Accidental removal | – Flush with saline<br>– Keep track open with balloon, PEG or Foley catheter | 4% |
| Peritonitis | If pain, stop feed, arrange PEG-O-Gram, inform seniors | 2% |
| Aspiration pneumonia | | 1% |

## PERCUTANEOUS ENDOSCOPIC GASTROSTOMY (PEG) FEEDING

PEG is an alternative method to provide direct tube enterostomy feeding (Fig. 13.1). The technique involves insertion of a guide-wire through the stomach wall under local anaesthesia and endoscopically guided insertion of the PEG through the abdominal wall over the guide-wire. PEG feeding is particularly useful following head injuries, for oropharyngeal malignancy and for some forms of intestinal failure. It is not suitable for patients with intestinal obstruction, ascites or undergoing peritoneal dialysis. There are complications specific to PEG feeding (Table 13.3).

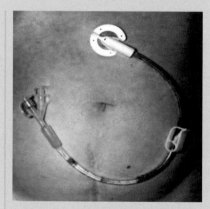

Figure 13.1 **PEG tube for enteral feeding.**

## INITIATION OF ENTERAL FEEDING

A useful regimen in patients with an otherwise normal gut is to start at 20 ml/h for 6 hours, then increase by 20–30 ml/h and repeat the process. If gastric tubes are used, aspiration to assess the gastric residual can be performed before each increase, bearing in mind that some aspiration of gastric contents is normal. If the volume aspirated is less than 200 ml, this is generally returned to the stomach and the rate of feeding increased. If there is reason to believe that absorptive capacity will be a problem (for example, with prolonged disuse leading to villous atrophy or significant small bowel resection), the progression to full feeding may need to be much more gradual to prevent diarrhoea. Diarrhoea is one of a number of potential complications of all modes of enteral feeding (Table 13.4).

## TABLE 13.4

### COMPLICATIONS OF ENTERAL FEEDING

**Related to intubation of gastrointestinal tract**
- Fistulation
- Wound infection
- Peritonitis
- Displacement and catheter migration (including small bowel obstruction)
- Blockage of tube

**Related to delivery of nutrient to gastrointestinal tract**
- Aspiration and hospital-acquired pneumonia (especially if feed contaminated)
- Feed intolerance
- Diarrhoea

On a daily basis, surgeons should review the indications for feeding, nutritional requirements and the chosen route of supplementation. In particular, patients receiving parenteral nutrition should be switched to the enteral route as soon as gut function returns or underlying abdominal problems settle.

## MANAGEMENT OF DIARRHOEA

Diarrhoea can be a major problem in enterally fed patients and can be multifactorial. The commonest identifiable cause is concomitant administration of antibiotics, which leads to de-population of the normal gut flora, and also has a direct irritant effect. If the antibiotics can be stopped, the diarrhoea will usually resolve rapidly. Other contributory factors include loss of intestinal absorptive surface because of villous atrophy or resection. The effect of villous atrophy can be minimised by maintaining

a degree of enteral intake or introducing it soon after surgery, even if it falls well short of meeting total nutritional needs. It is important to rule out infection with *Clostridium difficile* or other bacterial dysenteries before treating with agents to slow gut transit. Such agents include loperamide, codeine or kaolin–pectin mixtures, and can be very effective, especially after extensive small bowel resection.

A protocol for the management of enteral nutrition associated diarrhoea is given in Fig. 13.2.

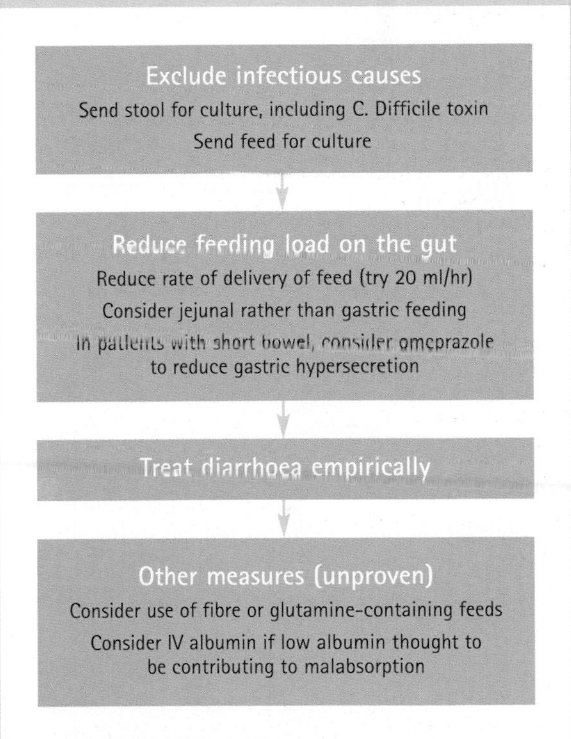

Figure 13.2 Protocol for the management of enteral nutrition associated diarrhoea.

# PARENTERAL NUTRITION

Total parenteral nutrition (TPN) can be defined as the provision of all nutritional requirements by the intravenous route alone. NICE has produced guidelines on artificial nutritional support, emphasising the careful balance between potential risks and benefits in all patients. Surgical conditions associated with a need for TPN are listed in Table 13.5, though the only absolute indication is the presence of an enterocutaneous fistula.

If possible, a dedicated line should be used for the administration of TPN. Due to the high osmolality of the mixture, TPN must be given into a central vein. In many hospitals the peripheral route to a central vein (peripherally inserted central line or PICC line) is preferred. Alternatively, a central line is inserted in the subclavian vein, or internal jugular vein tunnelled to an infraclavicular position to reduce infection risk. The tip of the line should be screened into the distal superior vena cava because this promotes maximal mixing of the feeding solutions with venous blood, reducing the risk of catheter-associated thrombosis. Intravenous feeding via the femoral vein should be avoided because of the high incidence of line infection and other catheter-related complications. The exit site should be protected carefully with an occlusive dressing and full aseptic technique used when dressings are changed or the line handled.

## TABLE 13.5

### INDICATIONS FOR TOTAL PARENTERAL NUTRITION IN SURGICAL PATIENTS

**Critical illness**
- Where enteral feeding is not established within 5 days

**Obstruction of the gastrointestinal tract**
- For example, patients with proximal small bowel obstruction which cannot be immediately relieved and who require pre-operative feeding

**Short bowel syndrome**
- Patients with < 300 cm of functional small intestine usually require at least temporary TPN. In many cases, adaptation will eventually permit enteral nutrition alone. Patients with less than 100 cm of small bowel generally require life-long TPN

**Proximal intestinal fistulae**
- May facilitate fistula closure. Use where enteral intake is restricted

**Refractory inflammatory disease of the gastrointestinal tract**
**Inability to use the gastrointestinal tract for other reasons**
- For example, pancreatitis with pseudocysts/ abscess where enteral nutrition is not tolerated

## COMPLICATIONS ASSOCIATED WITH TPN

The potential severity of line sepsis should not be underestimated and a high degree of suspicion maintained if a patient develops signs of sepsis or unexplained clinical deterioration. When a multi-lumen catheter has to be used, one channel should be preserved solely for TPN. The most common source of infection in catheter-related sepsis is the hub of the catheter. Strict aseptic technique is essential at all times, cleaning the hub with chlorhexidine whenever used. Three-way taps should not be used when TPN is being infused, and unless catheter-related sepsis is suspected, the catheter should not be used to draw blood samples.

Other catheter-related complications and metabolic disturbances associated with TPN are shown in Table 13.6. Also, fluid overload can occur, usually as a result of inappropriate continuation of other intravenous fluids, and electrolyte disturbances are relatively common though are usually predictable and preventable.

Refeeding syndrome is a rare and often preventable complication, which causes confusion and weakness associated with electrolyte disturbances. Criteria for determining people at high risk of developing refeeding problems have been devised by NICE, including low BMI, duration of reduced intake, degree of weight loss and electrolyte abnormalities. In those at risk, feeding should be introduced gradually over 48-72 hours.

---

### TABLE 13.6

#### COMPLICATIONS ASSOCIATED WITH THE PROVISION OF TPN

**Catheter-related**
- Mechanical – blockage, central vein thrombosis, migration, fracture, dislodgement
- Infective – exit-site infection, line sepsis, infective endocarditis

**Metabolic**
- Hyperglycaemia – too much glucose infused. Occasionally seen in severe sepsis, treat with insulin
- Deranged liver function – cause unclear but may relate to biliary stasis, enzyme induction from amino acid imbalance and excessive calorie administration, with fat deposition in liver
- Hypoglycaemia – too rapid cessation of glucose infusion
- Hypertriglyceridaemia – too much lipid infusion
- Hyperchloraemic acidosis – too much chloride in nutrient solution

# ADVANCED NUTRITIONAL THEORY AND PRACTICE

## METABOLIC RESPONSE TO STARVATION, INJURY AND SEPSIS

Malnutrition in surgical patients may occur from starvation due to fasting, but surgery and sepsis also cause a systemic metabolic response that contributes significantly to the clinical picture and to nutritional management.

### Feeding and fasting

In health, feeding replenishes fuel stores and the oxidative metabolism of fuel generates energy for metabolic processes. The normal daily resting energy expenditure of a 70 kg man is approximately 1800 kcal. The brain uses carbohydrate as its sole fuel in the fed state and requires approximately 100 g of glucose per day. Any glucose not consumed by the brain is used to restore liver carbohydrate stores (glycogenesis) and the rest is converted to fat (lipogenesis).

Amino acids are used to replenish those lost in the normal daily turnover of protein (including skeletal and cardiac muscle, liver and intestinal structural proteins and liver export proteins such as albumin) while the rest are metabolised in the liver, converting the carbohydrate component into fuel (gluconeogenesis) and the nitrogenous component to urea for excretion.

Lipid is stored primarily as triglyceride within adipose tissue. Lipid cannot be directly converted into either amino acids or glucose.

The hormonal environment associated with recent feeding (high insulin levels and low glucagon levels) allows the storage of nutrients as described above.

Fasting leads to a number of changes in the utilisation of energy sources within the body (Table 13.7). After a short (12-hour) fast, all of the food ingested during the previous meal is likely to have been utilised. The major source of glucose for the brain shifts to glycogen stored in the liver (of which there is approximately 200 g). This breakdown of glycogen to provide glucose (glycogenolysis) is facilitated by decreasing insulin levels and increasing glucagon levels. Though skeletal muscle contains a larger amount of glycogen (500 g), this cannot directly contribute to the provision of glucose for other tissues. Instead, glucose is converted to lactate within muscle, which is exported to the liver for conversion to glucose ('Cori cycle'). Glucose is also converted to lactate within haemopoietic tissues.

Muscle derives approximately one-third of its energy from the oxidation of glucose and the rest from the oxidation of fatty acids derived from the breakdown of fat in adipose tissue (lipolysis). Muscle protein breakdown begins to contribute amino acids (alanine and glutamine) for hepatic gluconeogenesis. After about 48 hours of starvation, approximately 75 g of muscle protein is being broken down each day. Glycerol and triglycerides from fat depots are used to make up the shortfall in energy requirements and fatty acids provide the main metabolic fuel for many tissues.

With more prolonged fasting, a series of metabolic adjustments develop in order to preserve body protein. For example, the liver gradually increases its capacity to produce ketone bodies from fatty acids. The brain adapts to use ketone bodies, reducing muscle breakdown by up to 55 g/day and preserving vital muscle and visceral protein. This is maintained as long as ketone body production persists, fuelled by the availability of fat stores. While absolute rates of protein breakdown decrease (in contrast to critical illness), the reduced anabolism which results from the lack of substrate leads to a net catabolism. These metabolic adjustments are associated with low levels of insulin and high plasma glucagon concentrations. A gradual decline in the conversion of inactive thyroxine (T4) to active triiodothyronine (T3) results in a fall in energy requirements to approximately 1500 kcal/day.

## TABLE 13.7

### METABOLIC RESPONSES TO FASTING

- Insulin levels fall
- Glucagon levels rise
- Hepatic glycogenolysis
- Muscle and visceral protein catabolism
- Hepatic gluconeogenesis
- Lipolysis
- Ketogenesis – sparing 55 g/day of muscle protein
- Fall in metabolic rate
  (typically to 1500 kcal/day)

*Metabolic responses to surgery*
Many of the metabolic responses to surgery, or injury in general, can be understood on the basis of the associated hormonal alterations (see Table 13.8). Release of noradrenaline, adrenaline, glucagon, growth hormone and cortisol occurs. Initially, plasma insulin levels fall but may later rise to levels in excess of those normally encountered for a given glucose concentration. The normal anabolic effects of insulin are impaired (insulin resistance). In addition, there

is a relative increase in glucagon concentration. The hormone response increases with the severity of trauma and its effect is to increase the availability of fuel for metabolic processes.

There is a modest increase in the metabolic rate to approximately 2000 kcal/day and lipid is the major fuel used for energy production. Muscle protein breakdown increases and glycogenolysis and gluconeogenesis result in an increased availability of glucose. This is used primarily by the brain, white blood cells and healing tissues. Glutamine is also released from skeletal muscle and, under conditions of stress, appears to be essential for the normal functioning of cells in the small intestine and immune system.

As the stress response reduces and insulin resistance falls, there is a shift towards a net anabolism, making up the lost reserves of protein and energy. This usually coincides with the resumption of eating and of increasing mobility, both of which are required to restore muscle mass.

## TABLE 13.8

### METABOLIC RESPONSE TO INJURY

- Modest rise in metabolic rate (and, therefore, energy expenditure) – typically 2000 kcal/day
- 'Counter-regulatory' hormone response – adrenaline, noradrenaline, cortisol, glucagon and growth hormone
- Resistance of tissues to effects of insulin
- Glucose intolerance
- Preferential use of lipid as energy source
- Exaggerated gluconeogenesis and breakdown of muscle protein, despite feeding
- Loss of adaptive ketogenesis

*Metabolic response to sepsis*

The changes in metabolism that develop with the onset of sepsis are complex and are an exaggeration of those described after injury (see Table 13.9). The key changes are a markedly increased metabolic rate (hypermetabolism) and rate of protein breakdown. There may be marked glucose intolerance with the development of a diabetes-like state. Despite this hyperglycaemia, glucose utilisation and storage are impaired and the septic patient has a greater reliance on fat as a metabolic fuel for energy production. There is frequently marked fluid retention. The rate of protein breakdown may reach 250 g/day. Muscle and visceral protein is thus consumed for the generation of glucose, despite the frequently elevated plasma glucose concentration. Although some of this exaggerated muscle protein breakdown might be due to the hormonal environment, the release of cytokines such as interleukin-1, interleukin-6 and tumour necrosis factor may also be implicated.

TABLE 13.9

METABOLIC RESPONSE TO SEPSIS/SIRS

- More marked increase in metabolic rate, hence energy expenditure (2200–2500 kcal/day)
- Exaggerated gluconeogenesis, protein catabolism and muscle wasting
- Marked fluid retention
- Insulin resistance common and may be severe

## ASSESSMENT OF NUTRITIONAL STATUS

Protein-energy malnutrition (PEM) often goes unrecognised in surgical patients, despite its prevalence and adverse prognostic implications. An assessment of the patient's nutritional status should form part of every physical examination. Gross degrees of malnutrition such as obvious wasting are easily recognised but more subtle degrees of deficit may not be, particularly in the obese patient. Body weight standardised to height as BMI is probably still the most useful measure of nutritional status.

Anthropometric measurements (*e.g.* measures of skinfold thickness and mid–arm circumference) allow estimation of muscle mass (protein reserves) and fat mass (energy reserves) but are often inaccurate, particularly in critically ill patients. Functional tests, including hand grip and respiratory muscle strength are predictive of the loss of muscle mass loss but have limited clinical use. Formulas to assess energy requirements, such as the Harris–Benedict equation, rely on poorly substantiated 'correction factors' for various clinical conditions such as sepsis or burns, and tend to overestimate energy expenditure. The most accurate way (albeit still with substantial variability) to assess energy expenditure in the clinical setting is by indirect calorimetry, using a bed-side 'metabolic cart'. This technique, which involves measurement of oxygen consumption and $CO_2$ production requires expensive equipment and is generally beyond routine clinical use.

Laboratory tests which are claimed to reflect malnutrition such as albumin principally measure how 'sick' the patient is, rather than measures of inadequate nutritional intake *per se*. For example, in simple starvation, serum albumin concentrations remain unaltered for nearly 6 weeks and begin to fall just before death. In contrast, in sepsis, the serum albumin concentration commonly falls to below 20 g/l within a couple of days or even hours, principally due to re-distribution into the interstitial space.

Laboratory investigations to look for the presence of associated trace element, vitamin and electrolyte deficiencies, however, may be of value. Measurement of standard electrolytes, along with magnesium, calcium and phosphate will enable demonstration of major electrolyte abnormalities. Interpretation of sodium and potassium balance can be difficult in critically ill patients, especially in the presence of large gastrointestinal losses (*e.g.* in association with an intestinal fistula or a proximal stoma), but they should be checked on a daily basis (see Table 13.10).

While an assessment of the degree of metabolic stress to which the patient is being subjected can be made, the most important step in nutritional assessment is to consider the need for nutritional support in every patient based on the underlying diagnosis, recent events and the likely time to restoration of adequate nutritional intake. Adequate nutritional intake does not automatically occur when the patient is first allowed to commence oral fluids!

## INTESTINAL FAILURE

Intestinal failure can be said to exist when the functioning intestinal mass of a patient is reduced below the minimal amount necessary for the adequate digestion and absorption of food. Like renal failure, intestinal failure is the end result of many different disease processes. It is also a continuum ranging from temporary mild dysfunction to complete and irreversible failure needing chronic 'replacement therapy'.

---

**TABLE 13.10**

BLOOD TESTS IN THE MONITORING OF NUTRITIONAL STATUS IN STABLE PATIENTS (IN THE UNSTABLE PATIENT, THE FREQUENCY WILL BE INCREASED)

**Daily**
– Full blood count
– Glucose (may need feeding and fasting samples)
– Urea, creatinine and serum electrolytes

**Weekly**
– Magnesium, calcium, phosphate
– Chloride
– Albumin
– Bilirubin
– Transaminases
– Gamma glutamyl transpeptidase
– Alkaline phosphatase
– Prothrombin time

**Twice monthly**
– Vitamin $B_{12}$ and folate
– Iron and iron-binding capacity
– Copper, zinc, selenium
– Pre-albumin, transferrin

At one extreme, intestinal failure may be an acute reversible problem (*e.g.* small bowel obstruction); at the other, a chronic condition resulting from an irreversible loss of gut mass (*e.g.* mesenteric vascular occlusion). Intestinal failure is a clinical diagnosis based on a history and examination, laboratory investigations and, in some cases, radiological investigations. Establishing a diagnosis of intestinal failure is important because attempts to provide enteral nutritional support alone are likely to be ineffective and early parenteral nutrition should be considered, possibly with referral to a specialised unit.

## SUMMARY

Nutritional support of the critically ill is a frequently neglected, but integral, part of the delivery of surgical care. Just as the support of the cardiovascular and respiratory systems of critically ill patients is based on an understanding of the altered physiology associated with disease, nutritional intervention is based on an understanding of the metabolic processes in the critically ill. The ultimate goals of nutritional support in the surgical patient are to ensure that the patient is optimally prepared for the stress of a surgical procedure and that recovery, even in the face of complications, is associated with minimal depletion of body stores. Use the expertise available to you on the surgical and high dependency wards, from nursing staff, dieticians and dedicated nutritional teams.

- think about nutrition in every patient
- assess status and nutritional requirements
- select the optimum route
- check that delivery is successful by monitoring the response.

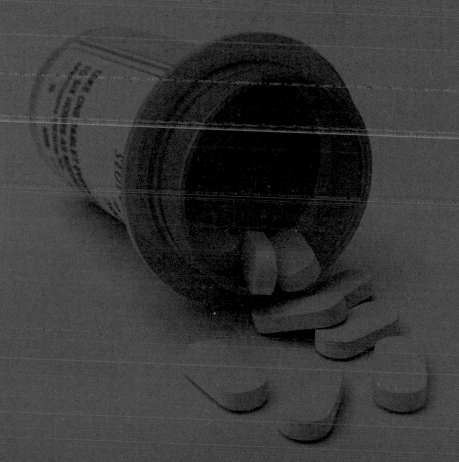

# 14

# Pain management

## INTRODUCTION

Nociception is the name given to the reception of a noxious or unpleasant stimulus and its conversion into an impulse transmitted through a sensory nerve. Pain refers to the perception of that sensation in the CNS and its recognition as unpleasant. Suffering is the emotional response that makes one miserable and is associated with the severity of the pain and its duration.

Society relies on doctors to provide relief of pain and suffering. It is important for all doctors to have a fundamental understanding of pain including how it is generated and perceived. As a member of the surgical team, you will look after patients presenting with primarily painful conditions and will encounter pain produced by surgical operations and interventions.

Safe and effective management of acute pain is an integral part of surgical practice. Although the physical status of the patient, the degree of trauma and the available techniques may be very different, the principles involved are similar whether the patient is recovering from major surgery on a general ward or being managed on an HDU or ICU.

Good quality analgesia is essential for humanitarian reasons alone: there are also compelling medical reasons for its provision. Inadequately controlled pain increases sympathetic outflow leading to an increase in heart rate, vasoconstriction and increased oxygen demand, particularly in the myocardium where it may contribute to ischaemia. It may impair lung function; abdominal and thoracic procedures almost always lead to impaired respiratory function because the pain induced by movement inhibits coughing and diaphragmatic function leading to atelectasis/pneumonia. The patient who has adequate analgesia is able to mobilise and this will reduce the incidence of deep vein thrombosis, improve respiratory function and improve general psychological well being.

It should also be recognised that pain postoperatively may be caused by a developing surgical complication.

However, a degree of pain is not always bad. Pain causes people to rest and protect injured tissue, preventing further damage and allowing healing.

# PRINCIPLES OF ACUTE PAIN MANAGEMENT

The realistic aim of pain relief is not to abolish pain in the postoperative period totally but to ensure that patients are comfortable and have return of function with a more rapid recovery and rehabilitation. There are several important principles relevant to the provision of good quality pain relief.

## PREVENT

The single most important step we can take in alleviating pain is to prevent the factors that produce it. Avoiding tension during surgical closure may help, as may preventing drains or tubes from pulling on sutures or relieving urinary retention.

The use of drugs preventing the development of pain is more effective than treatment of existing established pain. This is the concept of pre-emptive analgesia. In practical terms, this means that local anaesthetic drugs or other analgesic agents should be given prior to surgical trauma rather than afterwards.

## RECOGNISE NEW PROBLEMS

It is critical that trainee surgeons are able to recognise when a patient's pain has altered to a point where an alternative explanation is required. Any patient who has escalating analgesic requirements needs to be assessed with a high degree of suspicion (see Case Scenario 14.1). Ischaemia is a common trap, as are bleeding, anastomotic leakage and compartment syndrome. 'Breakthrough pain' in a patient who previously had effective analgesia should be treated as a surgical complication until proven otherwise.

## MANAGE EXPECTATION

The two most powerful forces in play during pain management are the expectation of the patient and that of the healthcare staff. If either believe that the patient will be in severe pain, the outcome will tend towards poorer mobilisation and poorer outcomes; if both believe the converse, the outcome is likely to be fewer complaints and more rapid mobilisation.

Pre-operatively, patients should be told to expect significant pain in proportion to their condition. They should also be told that pain can be controlled by various means and that they will not be allowed to suffer. If distressed by their pain, or if pain is inhibiting their breathing or their ability to cough, a change in technique will be required!

## SURGICAL CONSIDERATIONS

Upper abdominal incisions are associated with considerably more pain, more pulmonary

---

## CASE SCENARIO 14.1

A 75-year-old man has worsening abdominal pain 3 days after low anterior resection. He is requiring continued high-dose PCA morphine and is now nauseated and vomiting with a tender abdomen.
An anastomotic breakdown and collection in the abdomen needs to be excluded as the patient should be having decreasing analgesic requirements by this time. The nausea and vomiting may be due to obstruction not opiate. This patient needs a full clinical assessment to deduce the cause of deterioration and increased analgesia requirement.

disturbance and more difficulty effecting adequate analgesia than lower or transverse abdominal incisions. The choice of site and type of incision is therefore important in the sick patient who has limited respiratory reserve.

Laparoscopic surgery is considerably less traumatic and so less painful during the postoperative course.

Postoperative pain management will be aided by the use of local anaesthetic infiltration at the time of surgery or by specific local and regional anaesthetic techniques. Epidural infusion analgesia is the most commonly used of these techniques; other examples include caudal blocks for perineal surgery, intercostal blocks for cholecystectomy, and ilio-inguinal blocks for lower abdominal incisions. Upper and lower limb surgery can have major nerve blocks or plexus blocks to provide postoperative analgesia.

## THE ROLE OF THE SURGICAL TRAINEE IN THE MULTIDISCIPLINARY ACUTE PAIN TEAM

The provision of postoperative pain relief has always been hindered by confusion about whose responsibility it is to perform this function. Traditionally, postoperative analgesia has been prescribed by the anaesthetist, administered by the ward nurses and supervised by a junior surgical trainee. The Joint College Working Party Report on Postoperative Pain recommended that each major hospital should have a multidisciplinary acute pain team consisting of surgeons, anaesthetists, nursing staff and pharmacists. With increasingly sophisticated methods of analgesia being used, it is vitally important that the surgical trainee liaises with the other members of the team and is aware of protocols and guidelines relating to acute pain management in the hospital.

### PRACTICE POINT

*As the clinician likely to be contacted first in the case of a surgical patient becoming critically ill, the surgical trainee must establish if:*

(i)   *pain is related to a surgical complication;*

(ii)  *poor pain relief is contributing to the patient's lack of progress; and*

(iii) *the method of analgesia is contributing to the patients deterioration.*

## PATIENT ASSESSMENT AND MANAGEMENT

### IMMEDIATE MANAGEMENT

In the critically ill patient in pain, patient assessment is vital. It should follow the same CCrISP system of assessment as in any other circumstance.

*Airway*

Start at the beginning by checking that the patient has a patent airway. Over sedation secondary to opioid drugs may be associated with episodic airway obstruction. This is particularly marked in patients who are elderly, obese, have a history of obstructive sleep apnoea (OSA) or who have had surgery to the head or neck. It may be exacerbated by the administration of other sedative drugs such as benzodiazepines.

## PRACTICE POINT

*Episodes of airway obstruction and resultant hypoxaemia often persist for 2–3 nights after major surgery. Supplemental oxygen should be continued for at least 72 hours in high-risk patients recovering from major surgery who receive any form of opioid analgesia (including PCA and by the epidural route).*

### Breathing

Check the respiratory rate, pattern and depth of breathing. Is your patient's respiratory function impaired by inadequate analgesia? Can he or she cough and expectorate properly to avoid problems later? The rational use of opioid analgesia has always been limited by the fear of drug-induced respiratory depression. A much more common problem is the patient slowly slipping into respiratory failure due to poorly controlled pain which is inhibiting movement and the ability to cough.

## PRACTICE POINT

*Respiratory rate is a late and unreliable indicator of opiate-induced respiratory depression. Sedation levels are a more sensitive indicator of impending opioid overdosage.*

*Severe hypoxaemia may occur in the presence of normal or usually raised respiratory rates. Poorly relieved pain, particularly in upper abdominal surgery is a major cause of failure to cough, sputum retention and hypoxaemia.*

*Remember pulse oximetry oxygen saturations are not a good guide to respiratory function, only to oxygenation.*

In the assessment of the critically ill patient in pain, it is therefore essential to assess the adequacy and depth of the respiratory pattern as well as respiratory rate, and to check the patient's ability to cough. Investigations including ABG analysis and continuous pulse-oximetry can be useful adjuncts to clinical findings when assessing a patient's respiratory adequacy (see Case Scenario 14.2).

### Circulation

Tachycardia should not automatically be assumed to be caused by pain – there is commonly an underlying cause.

A persistent tachycardia or hypertension caused by inadequate analgesia may potentiate the development of myocardial ischaemia, particularly in the patient who is already hypoxaemic. A common clinical problem is the differential diagnosis of hypotension occurring in the post-surgical patient. This may be due to any cause of shock, from simple hypovolaemia due to inadequate fluid input or bleeding, through cardiac failure due to CCF, ischaemia and infarction or arrhythmias and septic shock. The patient may also be receiving epidural analgesia and this may cause added confusion as to the cause of hypotension, due to the relative hypovolaemia secondary to vasodilatation. Patients with sympathetic blockade are very sensitive to inadequate volume replacement and care must be taken in these patients to replace fluid losses immediately.

This requires meticulous attention to the maintenance of accurate fluid balance charts, measurements of losses from surgical drains and a high index of suspicion for concealed losses.

## PRACTICE POINT

*Persistent hypotension and tachycardia in the post-surgical patient may be due to any cause of shock. All types of shock need to be considered, investigated and excluded.*

*Epidural analgesia should not be assumed automatically to be the cause of hypotension.*

*Disability*
It is important to assess whether the method of analgesia is contributing to the patient's clinical deterioration. Particular attention should be paid to the patient's level of consciousness as decreasing conscious level is an early indicator of opioid toxicity.

## FULL PATIENT ASSESSMENT
*Chart review*
If pain relief is felt to be contributing to the patient's deterioration, the drug charts should be reviewed with the following questions in mind:
- is effective analgesia prescribed?
- is effective analgesia being given?
- is the treatment appropriate for this patient?

The recorded pain and sedation scores should be reviewed and the scores repeated (see below).

*History and systemic examination*
The contribution of pain to the patient's general condition should be ascertained during your full patient assessment.

*Behavioural observations*
Assessment of pain by hospital staff is usually based on the patient's outward response, or 'pain behaviour'. Verbal complaints, facial expression, restriction of mobility and changes in heart rate and blood pressure are used intuitively to build an impression of how much pain a patient is suffering. While these are often good predictors of pain, it is important to realise that, in some individuals,

### TABLE 14.1

#### PAIN SCORING SYSTEMS

| Verbal rating scale | Is your pain: 0, absent; 1, mild; 2, discomforting; 3, distressing; 4, excruciating |
|---|---|
| Numerical rating scale | Which number describes your pain: 0, no pain; 10, worst imaginable |
| Visual analogue scale | No pain to Worst imaginable |
| Functional assessment | Can you move? Can you cough? |

such assessments may be quite wrong and we may significantly under- or over-estimate the level of suffering.

*Severity scoring systems*
The effectiveness of assessment of analgesia will be vastly increased if simple reproducible pain scoring systems are used. These systems emphasise restoration of function by assessing pain scores during movement and when coughing. (Table 14.1.) Pain scores should be recorded when the patient is taking deep breaths, coughing and on movement otherwise the score may be falsely low.

## PRACTICE POINT

*Pain scoring in the patient recovering from major surgery should be as performed routinely along with measurement of cardiovascular and respiratory parameters.*

*Increasing pain scores should alert you to potential complications.*

*Investigations*
Investigations assessing respiratory function are frequently used when assessing the adequacy of analgesia. Serial ABG analysis and chest X-rays are often used to demonstrate trends in respiratory capacity and sputum cultures are essential when planning antibiotic therapy. Remember that pulse oximetry only tells you about oxygenation not overall respiratory function – the reading of saturation should be interpreted in the context of inspired oxygen concentration and respiratory rate.

*Decide and plan*
If pain relief is adequate and the patient is improving then continue and review. If pain relief is inadequate determine why:
- is it due to failure of the method of analgesia?
- is it due to incorrect implementation of the method chosen?
- is it due to the development of a surgical complication?

Pain relief should be considered as an integral part of the patient's total care. In certain situations, the method of analgesia may determine whether the patient has a smooth postoperative course or becomes critically ill. In a patient who has pre-existing chest disease, for example, the analgesic technique chosen when an upper abdominal incision is planned may determine whether a period of postoperative ventilation on an ICU is required or not.

## TECHNIQUES AVAILABLE FOR THE MANAGEMENT OF ACUTE PAIN

It is important for all those involved in the delivery of pain services to understand the range of techniques available. At one end of this spectrum is the administration of single analgesic agents, often administered orally, to a patient in mild discomfort. As the intensity of pain increases, there is a need for an increased response from those providing the pain relief. In some cases, increased analgesic requirements may be met by increasing the dose or potency of the drugs used. Other situations will demand the use of more sophisticated regimens. Combinations of methods and agents may be needed (multimodal therapy).

Alternatively, effective analgesia may require the use of sophisticated techniques, such as patient controlled analgesia (PCA) or epidural infusion analgesia (EIA). In all surgical procedures there may be appropriate local anaesthetic nerve/plexus blocks or simple wound infiltration with local anaesthetic drugs used to reduce pain.

It may be helpful to think of the increasing level of intervention required with increasing pain in terms of the WHO analgesic ladder. As a patient's pain intensity escalates, so does the level of support needed (Fig. 14.1, Table 14.2). When the situation improves and the intensity of the pain decreases, analgesic requirements will also decrease and a technique from lower down the ladder can be used.

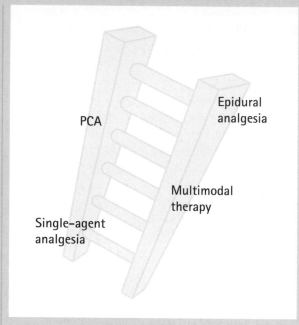

Figure 14.1 Analgesic ladder.

## TABLE 14.2

### PAIN INTENSITY ESCALATION AND MANAGEMENT

| Pain intensity | Management |
| --- | --- |
| Mild | Paracetamol or NSAID |
| Mild-to-moderate | Combination analgesic ± NSAID |
| Moderate | Oral opioid OR combination analgesic ± NSAID |
| Moderate-to-severe | Oral opioid + paracetamol ± NSAID |
| Severe | Parenteral opioid (i.v., i.m. or s.c.) + paracetamol ± NSAID OR epidural (local anaesthetic ± opioid) |

Combination analgesics are a mixture of weak oral opioid and paracetamol (see next page).

Opioids should only be administered by one route at a time – respiratory and other toxic effects from epidural opioids will be potentiated if oral, intramuscular or intravenous opioids are given concurrently. Such toxicity is potentially fatal!

## SINGLE AGENT ANALGESIA

Except in minor pain or discomfort, it is unusual for optimal analgesia to be obtained from a single agent or technique. If single agent analgesia is used, it will be more effective if drugs are prescribed and administered regularly rather than on an 'as-required' basis. All analgesic drugs can be given as single agents but are usually more effective when given as part of a balanced multimodal therapy regimen.

## MULTIMODAL THERAPY

It is often difficult to produce safe, effective analgesia with a single group of drugs. Better results with fewer side effects are achieved if combinations of drugs affecting different parts of the pain pathway are used. Such 'balanced analgesia' (multimodal therapy) usually consists of a combination of local anaesthetics, opioids and NSAIDs, and paracetamol.

## ANALGESIC AGENTS

*Paracetamol*
This is a very useful drug that has a high therapeutic index and very few side effects in normal dosage. It is toxic in overdose because it depletes the glutathione reserve of the liver and then damages hepatocytes. Paracetamol should be given regularly and can be administered by oral, rectal or, more recently, the intravenous route (as the pro-drug pro-paracetamol). It should form the basis of most in-hospital pain regimens.

*Non-steroidal anti-inflammatory drugs (NSAIDs)*
NSAIDs are increasingly used as part of balanced analgesia as adjuncts to opioid analgesia in an attempt to increase efficacy and reduce opioid side effects. Different preparations are available for dosing by sublingual, oral, rectal and parenteral routes. This group of drugs is unlikely to be chosen for the management of pain relief in the critically ill patient due to effects on haemostasis and renal function.

The COX-2 inhibitors are a newer subgroup; however, they are substantially more expensive than standard NSAIDs and accumulating evidence suggests that gastrointestinal side effects may not be substantially different and efficacy is no greater. They should not be used in patients with ischaemic heart disease.

*Opioids*

Codeine phosphate is an opioid with weak analgesic properties and, in randomised controlled trials, has an efficacy equal to paracetamol in adequate dose. However, it is profoundly constipating and may produce substantial nausea which limits its usefulness. It is often used in combination preparations with paracetamol.

Tramadol is a stronger opioid than codeine. It has many opioid-like properties but without the same extent of respiratory depression or the tendency to produce dependence. It does however have a marked emetic effect in many patients.

Although the bio-availability of morphine is quite low by the oral route, adequate effect can easily be achieved with dose titration. It carries with it all the usual potential side effects of opioids.

Patients with short-term needs or in transition to oral medication are best managed with morphine elixir; for chronic pain, a slow release tablet form may be most appropriate. Other opioids are also available orally or as slow release transcutaneous patches (fentanyl).

Opioids remain the gold standard of analgesia when a potent agent is required for severe pain. Morphine is the cheapest and most widely available agent. The principles discussed apply to all opioids, as do the toxic effects.

*Intravenous opioids – bolus doses*

Adequate analgesia is most rapidly achieved by an intravenous bolus dose, or repeated doses if the desired effect is not achieved with the initial dose. Often, boluses of 5 mg are given initially, followed by further increments of 1–2 mg until satisfactory analgesia is achieved. This may require surprisingly large doses; 20–30 mg is commonly needed in an average sized patient to produce good pain relief.

Once analgesia is achieved, i.v. dosing is commonly maintained by self-administration of further doses using patient controlled analgesia (see below).

*Intravenous opioid infusions*

Although opioid infusions can be very effective, respiratory and other side effects are common, and they should only be used in an intensive care setting. Intravenous opioid infusions are beyond the scope of the CCrISP course and will not be considered further.

*Intramuscular opioids*

The intermittent 'as-required' prescription of intramuscular opioid analgesia was the traditional form of postoperative pain relief. However, the use of 4-hourly intramuscular injections has repeatedly been shown to be ineffective in a high proportion of patients recovering from abdominal surgery and this technique has now been superceded by more effective methods of analgesia. It is also painful for the patient and has unreliable absorption in the hypovolaemic patient.

However a single one-off i.m. dose may allow you to relieve pain relatively quickly and safely while organising a more definitive analgesic regimen.

*Opioid side effects*

The limiting factor for use in the conscious post-operative patient is the emergence of side effects in a dose-dependent progression. All opioids exhibit similar effects, although the profiles of different agents may differ in the detail.

*Respiratory depression*

All opioids reduce the sensitivity of the respiratory centre in the brainstem in a dose-dependent manner. Even in therapeutic doses, the partial pressure of carbon dioxide (PaCO$_2$) will show an elevation from the normal value (5.3 kPa = 40 mmHg). A high normal (PaCO$_2$) of up to 6.5 kPa should be considered an expected consequence of using such drugs (as should constricted pupils) and is not a reason to stop using them. Both respiratory rate and tidal volume are affected by opioids. Respiratory rate is easier to measure at the bedside and it is extremely unlikely that dangerous respiratory depression will occur without a fall in rate below the normal range (12 breaths/min in adults).

*Sedation*

Decreasing level of consciousness carries with it the risk of loss of protective reflexes, especially those associated with protection of the airway (cough, gag and the ability to recognise imminent regurgitation). As unconsciousness deepens, airway occlusion may occur.

PRACTICE POINT

*A decreased level of consciousness is a medical emergency if the GCS is less than 8 due to imminent loss of protective reflexes and ability to maintain the airway.*

A low respiratory rate will usually improve by stopping administration of opioids. If the respiratory rate falls below 8 breaths/min, if the patient becomes hypoxic or is at risk from a decreased level of consciousness, small doses of the opioid antagonist naloxone may be indicated (100 mcg repeated until the desired effect is achieved). Be aware that naloxone may produce dysphoria, hypertension, tachycardia and the sudden and unwelcome return of severe pain if not carefully titrated.

Remember that the half-life for an intravenous dose of naloxone is short (approximately 15–20 minutes) and symptoms may re-appear.

*Nausea and vomiting*

This is a distressing and common side effect. It is dose-related and is potentiated by movement and when gastric emptying is already impaired. It is caused both by direct stimulation of the chemoreceptor trigger zone (CTZ) in the medulla and by gastric distention. Common anti-emetics available are ondansetron, cyclizine, metoclopramide and prochlorperazine. Dexamethasone may also help to relieve nausea.

PRACTICE POINT

*Nausea and vomiting may be due to a surgical cause rather than analgesic regimen or anaesthesia.*

PATIENT CONTROLLED ANALGESIA

The technique is based on the concept of the patient self-administering a bolus dose of morphine intravenously (usually 1 mg), after which the PCA machine will allow no further demands for a predetermined period – the patient 'lock-out' time. During this lock-out period, which is usually set at 5 minutes, the patient is unable to receive further doses. After the 'lock-out' time has elapsed, the patient is able to repeat the dose of analgesic drug if they are still in pain. In this way, the patient titrates their own level of analgesia, increasing demands when requirements are high (during physiotherapy for example) and reducing them when needs are lower or if they experience side effects.

## CASE SCENARIO 14.2

You review a 52-year-old man on the morning of the second postoperative day following a repair of an incisional hernia which had occurred in an old upper midline scar. Initial assessment shows the patient to be well built (95 kg), a little drowsy but adequately rousable. His breathing is rapid (24 breaths/min) and shallow and he cannot breathe deeply enough for you to hear his breath sounds well. He is sweaty, tachycardic (110 bpm) but normotensive and well perfused. A pulse oximeter showed $SaO_2$ of 88% initially – this has risen to 92% with mask oxygen at 6 l/min. He has a past history of smoking and mild chronic bronchitis. Review of his charts shows that 4-hourly morphine 10 mg has been given for analgesia.

You think that he is hypoxic, largely because of poor analgesia.

You increase the flow rate of oxygen to 12 l/min and ask for it to be humidified. The $SaO_2$ increases to 98%. The patient's conscious level improves and he affirms that he is in pain from his wound. It is 90 min since his last analgesia so you give a further 10 mg i.m. morphine and 20 min later he is more comfortable – auscultation now reveals reasonable air entry but some expiratory wheeze. Salbutamol (2.5 mg in 5 ml) is given by nebuliser.

Blood gases (on 12 l/min oxygen) show: $PaO_2$ 20 kPa ($FiO_2$, 0.6); $PaCO_2$ 7 kPa; pH 7.29; BE 0.4mmol/l; $HCO_3-$ 28mmol/l.

There is a mild respiratory acidosis and hypercarbia and an acceptable oxygen concentration. Note that the $SaO_2$ has not told you about the raised $PaCO_2$.

You arrange for review by the on-call physiotherapist and for a chest radiograph. After discussion with the pain team, arrangements are made for PCA to be established and you prescribe regular paracetamol 6-hourly either p.o or i.v, and p.o. or p.r. diclofenac 50 mg 8-hourly (having previously noted that he has normal renal function).

You review the patient at lunchtime. Repeat blood gases 1 h after physiotherapy show marked improvement. With continuous pulse oximetry, the oxygen flow is steadily reduced to 6 l/min. The patient is comfortable, breathing well and able to cough at will.

### LEARNING POINTS

- poor analgesia is common and has profound effects on respiratory and other vital organ function – 4-hourly prn opiates are often inadequate
- analgesic techniques are generally better at preventing pain than at rescuing a patient from marked discomfort with associated complications
- review the effect of interventions – re-assess your patient!
- a multidisciplinary approach can be very useful in pain management.

PCA is well accepted by patients and nursing staff, gaining high levels of patient satisfaction and providing good quality analgesia. The efficacy and safety of the technique depends upon the factors shown in Table 14.3.

## TABLE 14.3

### CHECK LIST FOR PCA

| | |
|---|---|
| Does the patient understand PCA? | Yes |
| Do the staff understand PCA? | Yes |
| Is the patient the only person pressing the button? | Yes |
| Is the pain responsive to opioids? | Yes |
| Is the patient receiving any other opioid or sedative drug? | No |
| Is the patient receiving a background infusion? | No |
| Is the patient being monitored appropriately? | Yes |

The major advantage of PCA is that it gives the patient control of their analgesia and greatly reduces the fear of unrelieved pain. It is also intrinsically safe; if the patient becomes sedated, they will administer no further drug, blood levels will fall, and they will recover consciousness. Sleep disturbance is a major problem with use of PCA. The requirement for regular dosing may prevent the patient having adequate periods of undisturbed sleep. Often, the pain is severe by the time the patient re-awakens and takes some time to bring under control.

PCA is unsuitable for patients who are confused or who are unable to press the demand button for physical reasons.

## EPIDURAL ANALGESIA (EA)
The most effective way of producing profound analgesia is to block afferent pain pathways by the use of epidurally administered local anaesthetic drugs.

*Insertion of the epidural catheter*
This procedure is commonly performed by the anaesthetist at the time of surgery. Both lumbar and thoracic approaches are used, the latter being commonly used to provide analgesia for both thoracic and abdominal surgery.

### PRACTICE POINT
*Many anaesthetists will not insert an epidural catheter if the patient has received a dose of anticoagulant prophylaxis within the last 12 hours. Consult with the anaesthetist if pre-operative heparin or LMWH are being considered.*

## ADMINISTRATION OF EPIDURAL DRUGS
The anaesthetist will have checked the position of the epidural catheter (ensured that it is in the epidural space and excluded accidental subdural or subarachnoid placement) by giving a test dose of local anaesthetic and will have established an infusion before the patient leaves the theatre suite. The infusion will usually be a mixture of a dilute concentration of local anaesthetic (bupivacaine 0.1–0.125%) with small amounts of added opioid (commonly fentanyl 2–4 mcg/ml). Combinations of drugs are administered for similar reasons to other routes – better analgesia with fewer side effects.

## CASE SCENARIO 14.3

8 hours after an uncomplicated right total knee replacement, you are asked to review a 59-year-old woman with ischaemic heart disease who has gradually become hypotensive (BP 80/40) and tachycardic 110 sinus rhythm.

You assess the patient and find her alert, comfortable and with acceptable perfusion. Continuous epidural analgesia is in progress, using a mixture of fentanyl and bupivacaine in standard dosage. There has been no chest pain, dysrhythmia or hypoxia (lowest $SaO_2$ 95%). Total volume in the drains is 750 ml, which the specialist nurse relates as 'average'. The wound is not soaked nor the leg swollen and the patient has received saline at 150 ml/h since returning from theatre. The epidural appears to be working well – the block is infra-umbilical, the patient can move her toes and is totally pain free. The infusion is running at 12 ml/h.

You conclude that the patient is hypovolaemic but cannot decide whether postoperative blood loss or vasodilatation from the epidural is predominant. The patient says she feels thirsty (a good sign of hypovolaemia). In either event, a fluid challenge is needed and you give 500 ml colloid over 15 min with little effect. During this time, a full blood count shows Hb 11.0 g/dl. You stop the epidural infusion.

Peripheral perfusion improves but blood pressure fails to respond. There are no signs of on going bleeding or narcotisation (which can occasionally occur). An ECG shows no acute change. Given the history of ischaemic heart disease, you are reluctant to give a further 500 ml fluid challenge so opt for 250 ml over 15 min. The BP begins to rise to 90/50 and the pulse drops to 100. You opt to give another fluid bolus of 250 ml colloid over 15 min and see the BP rise to 110/60 and pulse drop to 90. The epidural block is now decreasing and you decide to re-start the infusion at 6 ml/h and re-assess in 15 min continuing the maintenance fluids.

An hour later, the BP is maintained, there is good urine output indicating adequate renal perfusion and the patient is comfortable. You make plans to review the patient in 2 h.

### LEARNING POINTS

- hypotension associated with epidural analgesia is common – sympathetic blockade, peri-operative bleeding and loss of fluid into tissues or through insensible losses can all contribute – and investigations are needed to establish the cause
- postoperative bleeding must be actively considered and dealt with
- the need for treatment of hypotension due to the epidural alone depends on the level of the blood pressure, co-morbidity (especially cardiac or peripheral vascular) and the effect on end organs (urine output)
- all patients should be adequately filled with intravenous fluid – monitoring by CVP on HDU may be required in the patient with multiple co-morbidities.

The aim is to establish good pain relief with minimal sympathetic effects and no motor block. Infusion rates of 8–15 ml/h are commonly used. A functioning epidural gives outstanding pain control.

### Troubleshooting epidurals

The two most common problems are breakthrough pain and hypotension. Both may also be due to evolving surgical complications. Close co-operation between the surgical team and the acute pain service along with clear management protocols are essential.

### Breakthrough pain

This may be due to a problem with the epidural or the development of a new surgical problem. The patient should be fully assessed on each occasion. Help should be sought from the pain team if it is apparent that the epidural is not functioning. An increase in the infusion rate (often preceded by a bolus or 'top-up' dose) may be required or the catheter may require re-positioning.

### Hypotension

Hypotension is a relatively common problem with epidural infusions, particularly in younger patients and in those with higher level blocks. If hypotension is caused by the epidural, it is usually due to sympathetic block and consequent vasodilatation. As there are many other common causes of hypotension in the postoperative patient, the epidural must not be assumed to be responsible until other potential causes have been excluded. As always, when assessing the hypotensive patient with an epidural, use the CCrISP system of assessment to avoid missing other causes, especially hypovolaemia, bleeding, myocardial infarction and sepsis (see Case Scenario 14.3).

Once it has been established that epidural-induced vasodilatation is the cause of the hypotension, the infusion should be reduced and adequate fluid resuscitation should be undertaken to correct the relative hypovolaemic state.

## OTHER LOCAL/REGIONAL TECHNIQUES

There are numerous other techniques based on the use of local anaesthetic agents, which may be encountered in specific circumstances. These range from simple intra-operative infiltration of the wound to nerve blocks, plexus blocks, intrapleural infusions and so on. All have their proponents and specific indications, but all work on the principle of blocking generation or conduction of the noxious stimulus to prevent its being perceived as pain.

### PRACTICE POINT

*Patients may return to the ward with local anaesthetic infusions – these are severely toxic if infused intravenously.*

*This also applies to epidural local anaesthetic infusions.*

## CHRONIC PAIN

This is beyond the scope of this text, except to note that poor management of acute surgical pain may be one factor in the production of chronic pain and chronic analgesic dependence.

Paradoxically, the latter is more often produced by inadequate use of analgesics rather than over use, as is commonly believed.

## WHERE SHOULD SUCH PATIENTS BE NURSED?

For many reasons, including the provision of adequate postoperative pain relief, all patients recovering from major surgery should be nursed in an area with a high ratio of nursing staff to patients. Any ward designated for the care of patients recovering from major surgery should have enough trained nurses and doctors to care for patients requiring PCA or epidural analgesia subject to the following provisions:

1. The establishment of an acute pain service with named consultants responsible for the provision of postoperative pain relief.

2. Rapid 24-hour availability of designated doctors and resuscitation team.

3. A system for monitoring patients on a regular basis including pain scores, respiratory rate and sedation scores.

4. Protocols and an education programme for all staff for the detection and management of major complications.

5. Availability of continuous monitoring or transfer to an HDU or ICU for high-risk cases.

Provision of adequate analgesia is often difficult and complex in the sick surgical patient: consideration should be given to transferring such patients to a higher level of care.

## SUMMARY

- you are an essential member of the acute pain team, often being the first person called to a pain related problem
- when assessing the patient in pain, use the CCrISP system of assessment
- poor pain relief threatens the critically ill patient
- pain may be due to evolving surgical complications
- pain relief should provide comfort and restoration of function; analgesia should be assessed using reproducible pain scores and the ability of the patient to cough effectively
- multimodal therapy can dramatically improve pain relief and reduce side effects: remember the concept of the analgesic ladder
- PCA and epidural analgesia are very effective techniques but patients need careful monitoring and regular re-assessment to prevent problems
- be in regular contact with the acute pain team or your anaesthetic colleagues!

# 15

# Communication, organisation and leadership in surgical care

## OBJECTIVES

This chapter will help you to:

- understand the importance of clear and effective communication in surgical critical care
- appreciate some of the barriers to communication and ways of overcoming these
- develop an increased awareness of the leadership role, which the surgical registrar plays in the surgical team
- appreciate the value of personal and team organisation in facilitating this
- understand how people normally deal with adverse events and appreciate the frequency with which serious traumatic events can lead to stress reactions.

It is a self-evident fact that being an effective communicator is a vital skill for all surgeons. The way care is provided and the expectations of patients and relatives have changed markedly in recent times, posing new and challenging issues for surgical teams. Large numbers of people, coming from different aspects of the healthcare professions are now involved in the care of a single patient and this process needs to be actively managed by the surgical consultant and his or her team, who have ultimate and continuing responsibility for each individual patient. Patients and relatives, quite rightly, expect good outcomes from surgical interventions and expect to be kept informed about details of their care at each stage. It is vitally important to understand patients' expectations from the outset so that all concerned can understand what a realistic outcome for that patient may be. It is easy to make assumptions of what other people think and believe, which often reflects one's own beliefs rather than the reality for that individual. Many problems arising in surgical care are the result of poor communication, often serial, rather than a lack of knowledge or an incorrect decision. There is evidence to suggest that adverse outcomes, iatrogenic injuries, failure to provide adequate care, mistakes, providing incorrect care or system errors are more likely to lead to litigation or complaints if there have been preceding communication problems. Other international data on litigation have shown adverse outcomes occurring in 3.7% of admissions with 1 in 4 (1% of total) due to negligence. However, two out of three claims come from patients with no adverse outcome or an adverse outcome not due to negligence. Another study has shown that only 3% of patients who suffered negligence filed a lawsuit. Reasons given for instigating litigation include a desire to correct apparent deficient standards of care, to find out what happened and why, to enforce accountability and to gain compensation for accrued and future costs. A further study has shown that 70% of litigation is related to poor communication, citing feelings such as desertion, devaluation, lack of information and lack of understanding. In one study, over half of patients who commenced litigation claimed that they were so unimpressed by the doctor that they wanted to sue him/her before the alleged event occurred.

For the surgical team to function at its best, and thereby stand any chance of delivering optimum levels of care consistently, there must be good communication, organisation and leadership within the immediate team and with others. To achieve this, you need to understand some aspects of the ways in which people function under these circumstances, to learn to communicate better and to think about the ways in which you can contribute to the overall functioning and well-being of your team. Consider, for a moment, the range of tasks and scenarios you might face as a busy surgical registrar on call over a weekend, where communication, leadership and team skills are essential to a successful outcome. Having considered these skills, refer to Table 15.1 for a list of examples.

# COMMUNICATION

Communication matters – not just with the patient and relatives but also with colleagues. It is important to be able to communicate effectively for many reasons:

- to elicit and to provide information quickly and accurately. Especially in the critical care setting, the quality and efficiency of this aspect of communication (data transmission) is important
- to be able to respond to psychological and emotional issues in colleagues, patients and relatives (empathy, understanding and emotional support). This may contribute to improved outcome and will improve satisfaction ratings and reduce complaints
- to be aware of the possibility of tension or distress building up within the team and to know how to respond to this. Your team will not work well when it carries this type of burden.

A comprehensive account of basic communication skills is outside the remit of this chapter, although certain relevant communication skills are discussed and practised on the CCrISP course. You should develop an awareness of basic communication skills including: the appropriate use of open, focused and closed questions; knowledge and avoidance of leading and multiple questions; knowledge of and methods to overcome responses such as denial and blocking; understanding and use of empathic statements (see glossary).

| TABLE 15.1 |
| --- |
| COMMUNICATION SKILLS AND ORGANISATIONAL ISSUES TYPICALLY USED OR ENCOUNTERED DURING A WEEKEND ON CALL |

**Some tasks/processes**
- Informing patients and relatives of their condition and progress
- Obtaining consent for interventions
- Breaking bad news to patients or relatives
- Arranging investigations and ensuring the results are seen and acted upon
- Conducting ward rounds
- Speaking to senior colleagues
- Speaking to junior colleagues
- Booking cases for operating theatre and ICU/HDU
- Coping with multiple jobs
- Speaking to multiprofessional team members
- Dealing with emergencies
- Delegation and seeking help
- Identifying and treating patients in clinical priority

**Some skills**

| | |
| --- | --- |
| - Planning | - Leadership |
| - Active listening | - Mirroring |
| - Empathy | - Checking back |
| - Assertiveness | - Summarising |
| - Use of silent pauses | - Prioritisation |
| - Time management | - Delegation |
| - Avoiding aggressiveness | |

## WHAT ARE THE SPECIFIC COMMUNICATION PROBLEMS?

Often, surgical critical care takes place in an environment where background obstacles to communication are more likely. The patients are ill and frightened, and the staff are often over-busy. The patient may be unable to concentrate, especially if there is pain, severe illness or complications of medication. Equally, operational fatigue on the part of staff is also important. It is often easier for others to recognise the signs than for individuals to identify themselves. Signs of operational fatigue include loss of clinical sharpness and reduction in the quality of decision-making. Other obstacles to communication may include irritability and anger, high tension, confusion (most obvious in organic brain syndromes but may also occur in functional disorders), distress and tearfulness, and high expectations from patients and relatives but also from self and colleagues.

## SPECIFIC COMMUNICATIONS STRATEGIES

### The critical care setting

Strategies need to be targeted at the difficulties likely to be experienced. Critical care settings can be bewildering for patients and their relatives – often with a lot of unfamiliar equipment, sometimes with limited access to natural light. It is easy to assume that patients, relatives and doctors have a greater knowledge and experience of these environments than they actually have. It is especially important that at each stage, explanations are provided. These can be very simple tasks, such as explaining the role of a particular piece of equipment, an account of the next intervention or an explanation of where a specific issue fits

into the overall management plan. It can be helpful to try to predict what may happen and have a plan for the different possibilities. With regard to patients, especially the elderly, if they are in an environment with limited natural light, this may increase disorientation. Readable clocks or other ways of helping to overcome this are important. Especially where there is a degree of organic confusion, aids to orientation can be important, such as photographs of loved ones, and easy-to-read name badges.

It may be necessary to repeat both questions and explanations at different times. Being prepared to go back over the history after the immediate crisis is good clinical practice and may reveal issues previously unconsidered. It should be realised that many communication situations are not single episodes but rather a continuous process involving multiple episodes over time. Similarly, it is helpful to reduce fear by offering repeated explanations and using check-backs to assess that patient and relatives have understood. Patients can often only recall only small amounts of the information provided from a single communication episode.

### Breaking bad news

There is no perfect way to set out any communication process – what works well with some people in some situations can fail in others. However, some general principles are probably helpful. It can be useful to think about this is terms of what educators call the 'set'. This includes the environment where the communication episode will take place and who will be present. It also includes an introduction as to the purpose of the episode, the details of the episode itself and then a summary of the salient points of the discussion.

When speaking to relatives, it is important to ascertain that the patient has given permission for relatives to be informed of their condition. Understanding, if possible, intra-family dynamics can also help manage communications with relatives. For example, in some circumstances it may be felt necessary for the medical staff to talk to several family members together, while in others a family 'spokesperson' may be the best person to communicate with.

In terms of breaking bad news, an important principle is to be prepared to talk, and listen. The barriers to doing this may come from patients (or relatives if they are receiving the communication) or directly from us. Some things are hard for us to talk about but, in this setting, it is important to be able to tackle these. One way of starting such a conversation is to ask an open question such as 'what is your understanding of the present situation?', or 'what have you been told so far?'. In this way, you are giving the patient or relative the first opportunity to have a say and it may help you understand their expectations and how much they wish to be told. Some patients want a lot of detail, others only a broad outline. If you are unaware of the patient's expectations at the outset, you will not be able to meet them and you should not make assumptions. Starting in this way also gives you the opportunity to show that you are listening and to pick up on any verbal or physical clues as to the patient's or relative's underlying emotions. These can be subtle and you need to consciously look for them. You need to be prepared to use direct and understandable language. It is a great temptation to 'beat around the bush' in an attempt to soften the blow but it is important to say difficult, emotive words such as 'cancer' or 'death', should they be appropriate. It is often uncertainty that

people find difficult to handle; once they know what they are facing, they can start to deal with it and patients will often thank you for being frank and honest. Clearly, however, this can still be a delicate situation.

Attitudes have changed substantially in the last two decades but the work of John Hinton in the 1970s with people who had terminal illnesses remains instructive. He found that, in an in-patient unit, though staff believed that only a small minority of patients knew of their diagnosis and prognosis, a substantial majority had a very good understanding. This knowledge was acquired in various ways, including overhearing bedside conversations or reading case files. They were able and willing to share this with Hinton in a way that they had not done with the other staff. Importantly, when asked why they did not discuss their knowledge with staff, patients often indicated that they did not want to cause the staff distress. In other words, patients chose silence partly to protect the staff working with them. From this, the concept arose of being prepared and able to give the patient permission to talk about bad news.

To be able to give permission effectively requires good listening skills. Listening is an active process, interspersed with signs of encouragement. We all do this differently but should use attitude, facial expression or verbal acknowledgements to show interest and encourage further disclosure.

The use of empathic statements can be a straightforward way of identifying feelings and indicating support. These are statements in which the interviewer tries to identify a current feeling such as sadness, anger or fear and then ties it to what has been happening, such as 'It sounds as if this news has made you feel more fearful than anything else'. This can allow the person to talk about feelings and it also gives the interviewer a chance to check if what he/she perceives is correct. There are different ways of responding to sadness, anger and fear, for example. In contrast, sympathetic statements such as 'I know just how you feel', should be avoided. It is very unlikely that you could feel the same and such statements can lead to aggressive reactions from patients or relatives.

The most important aspects of helping people talk about feelings are to allow time and space. The setting should be quiet and private. The interviewer should give a sense of having time to talk. Often it will not take much time (in general, more skilled communicators take less time than less skilled communicators) but it does require planning to ensure, for example, that discussions like this are not started a few seconds before a ward round or some other fixed event. There is evidence to show that if a person is left to talk freely that they will speak for between 40–80 seconds. Allowing them to do so will start things off on the right footing and help the patient think you care about their problem. Sitting down to talk to the patient is good not only from the body language point of view but gives the impression of more time being taken. In a study where a doctor, who was either sitting or standing, spoke to patients for a set length of time, the patients' estimation of how long the doctor had spent with them was doubled if the doctor had sat down.

Another aspect of communication to be aware of is the use of 'mirroring'. The doctor mirrors what the patient is doing in terms of their tone and speed of speech, and their body language. For example, if a patient is sounding timid and scared, using a similar tone may convince the patient that they are being listened to and dealt with appropriately. If they are leaning forward, you should lean forward. It is not suggested that everything a patient does should be mirrored but doing the opposite to what the patient is doing can send a message that you are not listening or concerned about them.

A further issue for more junior doctors in particular is the way they handle their own uncertainties. In general, patients want definite statements and guarantees of outcomes. Clearly, there is much uncertainty surrounding surgical outcomes and you need to be able to appear confident in your knowledge, yet not lead patients to have unrealistic expectations.

At the end of the discussion, it is useful to make it clear that further meetings can be arranged and to give details of how this can be done. Giving the family a 'liaison' person can often provide reassurance that it should be easy to talk again. It is also important to document in the patient's notes that he or she has been spoken to, to provide a brief outline of what was said and to record any issues that may be relevant in the future.

*Medical mistakes*
Occasionally, people come to harm following a medical complication or a medical error. This raises quite different communication issues. In addition to breaking bad news, there is the additional matter of handling guilt feelings and fear of litigation. Again, it is not possible to make absolute statements but, in general, even in these situations, it is important to explain as fully as possible and, if an error has been made, to offer an apology. Not only is this in keeping with current thinking in the NHS but, since a sense of injustice often drives litigation, it is probably also a part of good risk management. It is important to be clear that one cannot apologise for the actions of others – you can state that you are

sorry to hear of their concerns/worries and that they are entitled to a full reply to questions/complaints. It is dangerous to apologise for an event that occurs outwith the individual doctor's control (*i.e.* by another doctor or member of staff). It is also important to realise that you should not criticise actions of others without very careful consideration. The GMC Good Doctor Guidelines stresses the importance of collegiality and it is very easy to comment on something without knowing the full details. Criticism of others is easy to imply by the most innocent off-hand remarks or ill-guarded body language. In certain cases, such actions can give the patient the justification in their mind to make a complaint or to seek legal advice.

*Working with colleagues*
Staff relationships are of particular importance in critical care settings. Not only does the work involve vulnerable and dependent patients, it also carries with it a lot of work-related emotional issues. It is easy for these pressures to translate into aggression and lack of respect. They may be made worse when inter-professional rivalries intervene or when people normally outside the unit are involved with particular patients.

Ideally, there needs to be some way for these issues to be dealt with on a team basis – identifying problem areas and finding supportive and effective ways of achieving change. Methods of achieving this cannot be prescribed but must vary with the precise situation. Deficient communication must be addressed, whether within or between professional groups, either by individual or group meetings, and formally or informally. These techniques often remain alien to the medical profession but can help greatly in the development of efficient and good-humoured units. Individuals

should also show respect in their own behaviour and learn how to use assertive rather than aggressive or passive interaction (see glossary).

## EVERYDAY COMMUNICATION IN SURGICAL CARE: ORGANISATIONAL SKILLS

Surgical training covers basic knowledge, operative skills and, through courses such as the CCrISP course, guidance in practical management of acute conditions. Only infrequently do trainees receive advice or instruction about the organisation of their practice. Regrettably, this is often discovered through trial and error.

In any training programme, there is a point where the surgical trainee begins to take increased responsibility for hour-to-hour management of patients, for critical decision-making about the requirements for treatment of emergencies, and to carry out major and emergency operations as appropriate. This has historically been on promotion to the registrar grade in the UK. Nowadays, the stage at which this occurs will vary but there is always a sizeable step-up in responsibility at some point in surgical training. Ultimate responsibility rests with the consultant in charge but no surgeon can expect to carry out procedures without sharing responsibility for peri-operative care.

Therefore, the senior trainee will often be responsible for the daily business ward rounds, reporting as necessary to the consultant. It is unlikely that the consultant will make a formal ward round every day so it is essential that the trainee actively manages the patients, looks for and identifies problems, makes decisions about management and contacts the consultant when appropriate. Initially, the trainee will communicate very frequently with his senior but, with training and experience, the scope for safe practice can and should expand.

For care to be delivered successfully in the context of a busy surgical practice, there are many facets of care during the working day including decision-making, investigations and operations. These do not happen automatically! As the trainee, you have to learn to conduct this orchestra of activity, and it is not always an easy task. To achieve success, you will need to organise yourself (and sometimes others), exercise a degree of leadership, communicate effectively and be able to make appropriate decisions.

To make decisions, you need information – and you get this from communication. As you train, you need to become aware of what information you do need and what information is largely superfluous to any critical decision. There is a balance to be struck between hasty and unfounded decision-making and un-necessary delay waiting for tests that will add little or nothing. Getting information takes you or others time and you need to delegate and organise appropriately. To be efficient, you need to time-table your business ward rounds such that key information is most likely to be readily available from nurses and house staff. You need to be prepared to circumvent blocks to your patients' progress. It may prove difficult to get old notes, get a certain test or opinion, administer a certain drug. At times you will need to be quite assertive on your patients' behalf to get what they need but you need to learn when to be, and when not to be, assertive. Building up good personal working relationships between other key members of staff will often help in this regard. The ward sister, the out-reach nurse, a clinical nurse specialist, the

emergency theatre sister and a friendly radiologist are just some examples. Think about the people who can make things happen for your patient and for you.

## ORGANISE TO MAKE COMMUNICATION EASY AND RAPID

To get the best out of a team, leadership is required – this requires a range of skills including ability, knowledge, personality, decision-making, appropriate humour, humility, acceptance of other views and firmness. All must be deployed at the right time and few, if any of us, possess all or even a majority of these attributes. You will need to work hard, praise and support your colleagues, admit when you are wrong or do not know and get timely help. Dealing with seniors is a whole skill in itself. Few consultants will not wish to be informed promptly about unwell patients but all will expect you to have assessed the patient, begun immediate treatment and arrived at some decisions including a provisional plan of action. The exception to this is the patient who clearly needs an immediate operation beyond your ability – for example, a collapsed patient with penetrating trauma – where the consultant will want a brief clear message and probably give you a brief and clear reply!

Clinically, you will need to lead by example – if you are not thorough, why will anyone else be? Re-assessing patients is probably the single most neglected skill – clinical patterns will emerge and diagnoses become obvious. With current working practices this is becoming more difficult and greater organisation is required for achievement. This underpins one of the basic CCrISP principles, of re-assessment after making decisions or instigating interventions. Utilise the support services available – good and experienced nurses can give you an enormous amount, particularly about how unwell a patient is.

Managing emergencies and deciding on the need for urgent surgery is difficult. Patients need a diagnosis and unstable patients need treatment urgently. Regrettably, patients do not magically improve between 2 a.m. and the 8 a.m. ward round – the emergency patient who fails to respond to simple resuscitation in the middle of the night needs a plan of action made then. This may involve conservative or operative treatment but lack of knowledge or an inability to conduct a particular operation is never an adequate reason for delay. Decision-making is active not passive!

Continuity of care is essential for patient well-being in critical illness. Junior doctor hours have changed but the need has not – the onus is now on the 'owning' team to pass on problems to the duty team, but also on the duty team to look for problems among the patients of all the surgical teams and to deal with them promptly. This poses the challenging communication task of a surgical handover when the responsibility of a large number of patients needs to be passed on to a different team. Within this patient group there will be patients who need specific interventions in a timely manner, patients who are getting better and do not need anything specific, patients who are at high risk of having problems, those who have not yet been fully sorted out and those who deteriorate unexpectedly. This latter group should be very small if the CCrISP principles of pro-active management, particularly for those who are 'slow' or fail to progress, are adhered to. A written handover list with a concise summary of each patient and a categorisation into one of the above categories is invaluable in this situation. This should be supplemented by a verbal reinforcement of which patients are giving cause for concern and some acknowledgement from the doctor receiving the handover that these patients have been identified and the responsibility accepted. Assuming the incoming doctor will pick up on these things instinctively is not acceptable.

Progressing up the surgical training ladder is a stressful but enormously rewarding time. You will very quickly develop new operative and patient management skills and begin to feel that you really are a surgeon. Organise yourself and your practice and communicate and listen effectively to make the learning process less stressful for all.

## COPING WITH ADVERSE EVENTS

Emotionally charged events are common in everyday life and particularly so in the critical care setting. This holds true for relatives and staff as well as for patients. Coming to terms with these everyday events is a largely automatic process. In simple terms, it seems to include having an awareness of the emotional reaction and somehow returning towards a normal balance. Traumatic stressors are events that produce intense pressure or tension; they are associated with the negative emotions of fear and sadness. In normal circumstances, these emotional reactions gradually decline and each subsequent recall of these feelings is rather less intense until eventually, as a new equilibrium is reached, the emotional reaction fades completely and the individual adapts.

Faced with events that are perceived to be especially traumatic, this adaptive mechanism may be overwhelmed. The initial emotional reaction may be so intense that the only viable reaction is to attempt to prevent or avoid (blot out) these painful feelings. This may be achieved by avoiding places or objects that remind the person about the trauma, or through suppression of emotions in general – 'emotional numbing'.

These defensive reactions will rarely be completely successful and the individual is left with painful intrusive recollections, which alternate with defensive avoidance. This cyclical reaction of intrusion and avoidance is the central element of post traumatic stress disorder (PTSD). It is possible that, as the emotions are suppressed because they are too extreme, they are not held in awareness and do not decline. The condition becomes chronic and may be frankly disabling. Stress disorders are not rare: some symptoms of PTSD are seen in the majority of patients who are involved in significant accidents and features occur in relatives of the victims and staff. Typically, patients may report recurrent and intrusive distressing recollections of the event including flashback episodes. These can be precipitated by cues, which symbolise or resemble an aspect of the traumatic event (*e.g.* hearing a car's brakes on TV or even driving past the hospital). The victim is likely to avoid thoughts or cues that activate memories of the event and may become withdrawn, detached or appear depressed.

Critical events are a significant cause of occupational stress for staff groups (including doctors) in this environment and this is important to recognise not only for personal and team well-being but also because operational fatigue and impaired performance may result. Awareness of stress reactions is the first step and the provision of appropriate support of colleagues and patients, largely through opportunities for discussion, will represent a significant advance in many settings. The initial aim is to provide a means for people to talk about a critical event, learning about some of the ways that people may respond and (usually) achieving an understanding that their own behaviour is within a normal range.

## COMMON PSYCHOLOGICAL DISORDERS IN SURGICAL CRITICAL CARE

So far, the emphasis has been on specific reactions to adversity but of course a wide range of problems may occur. Traumatic life events may trigger feelings of depression, anxiety or even relapse of certain psychoses. The assessment needs to cover the full range of psychological difficulties. In this section, brief reference will be made to four of these.

### ANXIETY

Mild feelings of fear, apprehension, sadness and emotional turmoil are very common in anyone admitted to hospital with a serious condition. In general, the approach taken by the clinical team can often determine the amount of distress experienced. A team that works well together, communicates well with patients and offers appropriate emotional support will reduce these difficulties, while dysfunctional teams will exacerbate the problem.

Assessment is likely to centre on asking appropriate questions about current feelings and enquiring into any associated autonomic symptoms of anxiety (*e.g.* tachycardia, raised blood pressure) which may mislead in the assessment of physical health. Sometimes, visible over-breathing (excessive, often irregular breathing) may be a clue to the presence of the chronic hyperventilation syndrome. This can present with a multitude of physical symptoms and is often associated with anxiety or depression.

*Major depression*

Depression is also a common condition and often unrecognised. It spans a wide range of severities and patterns of reaction. The core feature is a depressed mood, in which there is loss of pleasure and enjoyment, reduced interest, hopelessness and helplessness, and pessimism for the future. In addition, there are often biological features, such as loss of weight, impaired sleep with early morning wakening and a diurnal variation of mood – worst in the early morning. Finally, there may be evidence of a frank psychosis with mood-congruent delusions and hallucinations. These may include delusions of worthlessness or guilt, delusions of cancer, delusions of persecution (felt to be deserved), accusatory auditory hallucination. All these are in keeping with the primary disturbance of mood.

As a routine in the assessment of psychiatric disturbance, there should be an investigation of suicidal thinking. One of the ways of asking about this is to combine a permissions statement with a question. For example, if someone has talked about feeling very unhappy, they sometimes can not see much point in life. Then continue with something like 'I wonder if you have ever felt it would be better just to go to sleep and never wake up?' This can be followed by further questions about any suicidal thoughts, any suicidal plans (going into detail if needed) and any suicidal behaviour. In this way, the whole subject can be covered easily without causing excessive concern. There is no excuse for failing to ask about suicidal thinking in the presence of significant psychiatric disturbance.

## ALCOHOL DEPENDENCE

This is included as a reminder that alcohol problems are common (in general, about 1 in 5 people in hospital have significant alcohol-related

problems) and can cause complications in the critical care setting. The characteristic problem arises from withdrawal symptoms, which follow hospitalisation and enforced abstinence. These can include typical tremor, nausea, mood disturbances and confusion but may extend to delirium tremens and even convulsions.

## ACUTE ORGANIC REACTIONS

Variously styled as confusional states, toxic confusional states, deliriums, etc., these are short-lived organic disturbances characterised by confusion, clouding of consciousness (sometimes quite subtle), disorientation and often marked fearfulness. There may be delusions – often persecutory. Common causes include alcohol withdrawal and prescribed medication (*e.g.* analgesia) but they may also occur in the context of a wide range of medical conditions. Following assessment and correction of the ABCDs of the initial assessment, further evaluation is centred on the cognitive state – ability to attend and retrieve, awareness of environment, etc., and on the possible causes which also require full assessment. This is an organic disorder in the psychiatric classification because it is always secondary to some physical dysfunction. It is likely to be made worse by a disorientating environment and by a failure to offer frequent and repeated explanations.

## WHEN TO REFER TO A PSYCHIATRIST?

To some degree, this depends on the capacity and engagement of the local psychiatric service. However, there are clear indicators for referral, which are important to outline. First, there is the situation where the diagnosis is uncertain and especially where there may be a psychiatric component. Somatisation disorder and

Munchausen's syndrome are extreme examples but there are often complex interactions between physical and psychological processes which may require assessment. It is important in these situations to make positive psychiatric assessments rather than assumptions based on the absence of signs of physical disorder.

There are situations where either the severity of the psychiatric condition or level of danger associated with the condition make referral both appropriate and often urgent. This might be following, for example, deliberate self-harm or the development of persecutory beliefs in an acute organic reaction leading to thoughts of murder.

One situation in which referral is often considered is in relation to consent. Psychiatrists have special knowledge of the legislation to do with consent to treatment for psychiatric illness. The relevant legislation has much less to say about consent to treatment for physical illness and common law principles usually apply. Nonetheless, as long as a referral is not made with overoptimistic expectations, it may still be useful to discuss difficult cases where consent is withheld as this is an issue which is more common in psychiatric practice.

## SUMMARY

This chapter cannot provide a comprehensive account of the field but perhaps it will help to highlight those areas where further learning is required. This learning is not readily available in text books but can be gained with experience. It does require insight and reflection on the part of the individual, the latter skill being easily neglected in a busy surgical environment. Communication skills are especially important as they help to make practice more effective and efficient. More can be achieved in less time. It is important to look at patients, relatives and staff groups and understand the ways in which we cope with the everyday workload, with adversity and how these mechanisms can be overwhelmed at times of crisis.

# GLOSSARY

Most clinicians could improve their communication skills and surgeons are certainly no exception. The glossary outlines some principles about which you may wish to read further. The specific skills cannot be summarised in a short glossary but are included in most books on communication.

## BASIC COMMUNICATION SKILLS

In this section, some of the terminology will be explained. It is useful in data gathering to use an appropriate range of open, focused and closed questions. In taking a history, the open question 'Is there anything else?' is useful as a final question.

> Open questions can take a wide range of responses, e.g. 'What is the main problem?' Focused questions can take a limited range of responses, e.g. 'Which is the worst pain today?' Closed questions must be answered 'yes' or 'no', e.g. 'Is the pain in the knee the worst pain that you have?'

Some questions are likely to produce misleading answers. A leading question expects a particular response and this may be given even if it is wrong. Multiple questions are common in checklist approaches to the history but the answer given may only relate to the final item in the list – again misleading.

> A leading question expects a particular answer, e.g. 'The pain is worst at night, isn't it?'
>
> Multiple questions include a list, e.g. 'Do you have problems with chest pain, shortness of breath or ankle swelling?' This might attract the answer 'no' which to the patient might be 'no' to ankle swelling and to the doctor might be 'no' to the three items together.

There is a skill to checking back – being prepared to check that you have the right understanding – or using a summary of the main features as a way of confirming the history with your patient.

There is also a skill to sharing a problem. If you do not know how to handle something in an interview, sometimes the best thing is to own up. For example:

> 'I have a feeling that you are upset but I am not sure what has caused it. Is it OK to ask you about it?'
>
> 'My problem is that I only have 5 minutes before I have to go to theatre. I really need to ask you about something. Is that alright?'

Finally, perhaps the most useful of the active steps in understanding emotional reactions is the empathic comment. This is a statement identifying an emotional reaction, e.g. 'That must have made you feel very frightened'.

In making this statement, a lot of care must be exercised to listen to what is being said and not simply to assume that everyone will experience fear, anger, sadness, etc. in specific situations. It is useful as a way of checking back on emotions but, more importantly, it communicates that you can appreciate at least some of what your patient is feeling. This can be a very powerful intervention and should be a skill available to all doctors.

*Blocking*
Not facing an issue. For example, a patient asks 'are there any complications with this operation' and the surgeon replies 'don't you worry, it'll all be fine'. Another example is a doctor telling a patient they have cancer and the patient says 'it can't be cancer, I feel too well'.

*Mirroring*
Reflecting what the patient is saying in terms of tone of voice and body language. For example, if a patient is talking softly and timidly, reply in similar tones. If a patient is sitting leaning forward, do the same. Doing the opposite (anti-mirroring) can adversely affect interactions.

## ASSERTIVENESS, PASSIVITY AND AGGRESSION
In being assertive, communication allows each person to express their honest opinions without needlessly hurting the other person. In being passive, honest opinions are suppressed.

Aggression involves the use of excessive force or power causing needless suffering. This can be active aggression (*e.g.* violent, insulting speech) or passive aggression (*e.g.* emotional manipulation).

Assertiveness is, therefore, usually the preferred option. In general, assertive statements contain the pronoun 'I' whereas aggressive statements more often include the pronoun 'you', for example, 'I feel that the patient would be better helped by this approach' versus 'You are incompetent and have got this all wrong'.

# 16

## Assessment of surgical risk and peri-operative care

**OBJECTIVES**

This chapter will help you to understand:

- the importance of assessing peri-operative risk
- the factors that contribute to increased surgical risk
- the peri-operative management of diabetes.

Co-morbidity increases the risk of surgical procedures and minimising that risk is vitally important to improve the individual outcome. Risk assessment is also important in terms of outcome measures for comparative audit. Simple scales, such as the American Society of Anesthesiologists (ASA) grading system, are open to varied interpretation among experienced medical assessors, while more complex systems such as the POSSUM score, are too complex for most daily clinical applications.

Co-existing diseases can complicate even a simple operation and increase morbidity and mortality. The level of care required needs to be anticipated with consideration given to transfer to units with appropriate facilities and/or to gaining disease-directed expertise to advise on pre-operative optimisation and peri-operative management of individual co-morbidities.

The concept of a 'high-risk' patient is generally understood but the key is to recognise the factors contributing to that perceived risk and repeatedly (re)assessing these patients throughout their stay in hospital to minimise the risk of developing complications.

Many of the factors that increase surgical risk are covered elsewhere in this book. This chapter will discuss risk assessment in more detail and outline the specific effects of older age, obesity and, in particular, diabetes.

## CO-MORBIDITIES AND PERI-OPERATIVE CARE

Good surgical results reflect the quality of care. This depends on:

- surgical factors, relating to pre-, intra- and postoperative care
- patient factors, regarding disease presentation and pre-existing co-morbidities
- systemic factors that relate to the resources available for the treatment of surgical patients.

Pre-existing co-morbidity increases the risk of surgery. Anticipation of risk and risk factor modification are vital in attempting to reduce surgical morbidity and mortality. Co-morbidities most commonly associated with increased surgical morbidity and mortality are:

- cardiovascular (hypertension, myocardial ischaemia, cardiac failure and cardiac arrhythmias)
- chronic respiratory disorders
- anaemia
- diabetes mellitus
- chronic renal impairment
- obesity.

Emergency surgical conditions entail higher risk as do elderly patients because of the higher incidence of co-existing medical illness and a reduced physiological reserve.

# THE METABOLIC RESPONSE TO INJURY

An understanding of the metabolic response to injury is helpful in understanding how co-morbidity, particularly diabetes, affects peri-operative management and risk (see also Chapter 13, Nutrition). Metabolic responses to major injury, surgery and severe infection have similar mechanisms. The response occurs in two phases, referred to as 'ebb and flow'. The mediators and their effects for these responses are outlined in Table 16.1. The 'ebb phase' lasts 24–48 hours and is a neuroendocrine response to tissue injury and hypovolaemia. Cardiovascular reflex activity and inhibition of central thermoregulation are reminders of the 'fight or flight' response. Energy stores are mobilised to fuel the increased metabolic demand: plasma glucose concentration increases in proportion to the severity of the injury due to mobilisation of liver and skeletal muscle glycogen stores and the suppression of insulin release that inhibits the uptake of glucose into cells. Lipolysis is increased but fatty acid re-esterification within adipose tissue may be stimulated by the raised plasma lactate of severe injury or impaired perfusion of fat deposits. An early rise in hepatic protein synthesis and an increase in microvascular permeability are responsible for characteristic changes in plasma protein concentrations within 6 hours.

Survival beyond the first 1–2-day initial phase gives rise to the 'flow phase' of increased metabolic rate, principally due to muscle catabolism and resistance to the anabolic effects of insulin. The triggers for this are similar to the first phase but with increased energy consumption. The high energy source ATP is produced principally by glycolysis (an inefficient mechanism) and the lactate produced is reconverted into glucose in the liver in an energy-consuming process, thereby increasing hepatic oxygen consumption and blood flow. Protein catabolism predominates principally affecting skeletal muscle but respiratory, gut and (possibly) cardiac muscle are also affected, giving rise to problems with mobility, ventilation and enteral nutrition. There are concomitant increases in urinary excretion of nitrogen and creatinine. The increase in proteolysis provides amino acids as precursors for hepatic gluconeogenesis. Concentrations of the amino acid glutamine in skeletal muscle fall. Glutamine is an important fuel for cells of the immune system and it is a precursor for glutathione (a free radical scavenger); it has a role in nitric oxide metabolism and has also been implicated in the maintenance of the gut mucosal barrier which may be compromised after injury. Insulin resistance after injury refers to its anabolic effects; for example, hepatic glucose production, lipolysis and the net efflux of amino acids from skeletal muscle. These effects persist at plasma glucose and insulin concentrations that are inhibitory in uninjured subjects. Uptake of glucose into skeletal muscle is also reduced, an impairment that involves glucose storage rather than oxidation. The cause may result partly from counter-regulatory hormones cortisol, adrenaline and glucagon, although infusion in healthy individuals requires much higher plasma concentrations to cause insulin resistance than those found in injured or septic patients. So the effect of these hormones could be augmented by modulation of insulin sensitivity by pro-inflammatory cytokines: interleukin-6 in cancer patients, interleukin-1 in endotoxaemia and tumour necrosis factor in diabetes and obesity are all correlated with the degree of insulin resistance.

## TABLE 16.1

### MEDIATORS OF INJURY RESPONSE AND THEIR EFFECTS

**Counter-regulatory hormones**
(*e.g.* catecholamines [adrenaline], cortisol, glucagon, antidiuretic hormone)
- Breakdown of glycogen stores in liver and skeletal muscle
- Suppression of insulin release resulting in reduced uptake and oxidation of glucose

**Increased sympathetic nervous system activity**
- Lipolysis

**Protein metabolism**
- Increased hepatic synthesis (interleukin-6 induced)
- Increased microvascular permeability
- Raised plasma concentration of fibrinogen and C-reactive protein
- Fall in plasma albumin concentration

**Pro-inflammatory cytokines** (*e.g.* tumour necrosis factor-$\alpha$, interleukins ß, 2, 6 and 8)
- Mimic some responses, but plasma levels not universally linked to injury indicating autocrine/paracrine (cf. endocrine) function

**Interleukin 6 induction of prostanoids at the blood–brain barrier**
- Activation of the hypothalamus–pituitary–adrenal axis

# DIABETES MELLITUS

Diabetes is a state of impaired glucose tolerance caused either by absolute lack of insulin (type 1) or relative lack of insulin (type 2). In addition to the metabolic disturbance, micro- and macrovascular abnormalities cause retinopathy, nephropathy, neuropathy, coronary heart disease, stroke and peripheral vascular disease. Diabetics also develop cataracts and specific soft tissue disorders such as diabetic cheiroarthropathy as a result of exposure of the tissues to hyperglycaemia, causing accelerated irreversible biochemical and structural changes normally found in ageing. Improved glycaemic control in diabetes protects against these secondary effects.

Surgery can be hazardous to diabetic patients. The metabolic response to surgical trauma can rapidly lead to hyperglycaemia and ketoacidosis, especially in insulin-deficient patients. Poorly controlled diabetes accelerates catabolism and delays healing. Insulin and the sulphonylureas can cause severe hypoglycaemia in fasted and anorexic patients, which can be particularly dangerous during general anaesthesia. Assessment of fitness for surgery, pre-operative optimisation, an agreed management policy between specialists and ward staff and meticulous glycaemic control will greatly reduce the risks of operating on diabetic patients.

Some case examples will serve to illustrate the key management issues in patients with diabetes undergoing surgical treatment.

## CASE SCENARIO 16.1

A 33 year-old civil servant, admitted to the surgical unit for an open elective inguinal herniorrhaphy, is stabilised on thrice daily subcutaneous soluble insulin injection and is otherwise fit and well.

### HOW WOULD HIS DIABETES BE MANAGED PERI-OPERATIVELY?

Such patients have absolute deficiency of insulin and require an intravenous glucose-potassium-insulin (GKI) infusion to be instituted on the morning of surgery after an overnight fast and omission of the morning insulin dose. A protocol for GKI infusion is given in Table 16.2, though note that most hospitals will have their own local protocols.

He had an uneventful procedure under general anaesthesia on the morning list with hourly BM recordings showing good control with plasma levels of glucose between 5–10 mmol/l. Due to postoperative nausea and vomiting, the GKI regimen was continued overnight. By the next morning, he was able to eat and drink normally; the GKI infusion was discontinued and he had his normal morning insulin dose with his breakfast and was discharged home later that morning.

## CASE SCENARIO 16.2

A 67-year old retired coach driver was seen in the pre-admission clinic for work-up for an elective TURP for symptomatic benign prostatomagaly. He had been diabetic for 5 years and currently controlled with diet and glibenclamide.

### HOW WOULD YOU MANAGE HIS DIABETES?

Generally, type 2 patients well-controlled by diet or oral agents may simply omit their oral agents and breakfast on the morning of surgery. However, long-acting sulphonylurea drugs (*e.g.* glibenclamide) should be substituted by short-acting ones (*e.g.* glicazide) some days before surgery to reduce the risk of hypoglycaemia. Blood glucose should be monitored closely in the peri-operative period and persistent hyperglycaemia should be treated with a GKI infusion. If the patient is in a steady state, the GKI infusion will maintain satisfactory glycaemic control and prevent hypokalaemia. GKI bags must be changed if glucose levels are unsatisfactory. Alternatively, insulin may be given as a variable rate intravenous infusion according to a sliding scale (Table 16.3), which provides greater flexibility.

## TABLE 16.2

### PROTOCOL FOR GLUCOSE–POTASSIUM–INSULIN (GKI) INFUSION

**For stabilised patients only**

For intravenous infusion use 500 ml of 10% dextrose containing 15 U of soluble insulin (*e.g.* Actrapid) and 10 mmol of KCl
- infuse at 100 ml/h
- check blood glucose every hour
- check $K^+$ every 6 h and adjust accordingly

If blood glucose falls to < 5 mmol/l discard existing bag and replace with 10 U of soluble insulin and 10 mmol of KCl

If blood glucose rises to > 10 mmol/l discard existing bag and replace with 20 U of soluble insulin and 10 mmol/l KCl

Lower or higher insulin doses are sometimes needed

Check plasma $K^+$ every 6 h and adjust accordingly

This regimen is only for patients with stable and well-controlled diabetes; it should be started on the morning of surgery after an overnight fast and continued until the patient can eat and drink normally

## TABLE 16.3

### AN EXAMPLE OF SLIDING SCALE INSULIN INFUSION

This is for intravenous use in unstable patients frequently with hyperglycaemia. 50 U of soluble insulin is added to 50 ml of 0.9% isotonic saline giving a 1 U/ml solution for delivery using a syringe driver
- hourly monitoring of blood glucose concentration is mandatory
- start infusion at 6 U/h until the glucose level begins to fall
- subsequently, titrate so that blood glucose falls by 3–4 mmol/l each hour
- most patients need 1–3 U/h and this usually becomes clear after 3–4 hours of glucose monitoring

A typical sliding scale would be:
- blood glucose < 5 mmol/l, give 0.5 ml/h
- blood glucose 5–10 mmol/l, give 2.0 ml/h
- blood glucose > 10 mmol/l, give 4.0 ml/h.

## CASE SCENARIO 16.3

A 66-year-old woman was admitted from A&E with a 6-day history of feeling unwell, with immobility and discharge from the right foot. She had been diabetic for 7 years treated with diet, glicazide and metformin. Examination revealed discharge from the instep, a necrotic heel and cellulitis extending across the ankle into the lower leg. Her pulses were all palpable, but there was diminished pedal sensation. Her Hb was 11.1 g/dl, white count 18.6 x 10⁹/l, blood glucose 24 mmol/l, potassium 5.8 mmol/l, urea 9.0 mmol/l and creatinine normal.

### HOW WOULD YOU MANAGE THIS PATIENT?

She should be managed as per the CCrISP protocol, with immediate attention to the ABCs. Her diabetes is out of control. An intravenous insulin infusion according to a sliding scale (Table 16.3), with hourly monitoring of the blood glucose and 3–4-hourly potassium estimation (Table 16.4) is appropriate. She requires resuscitation with intravenous 0.9% saline until she has been stabilised, and her glycaemic and potassium control optimised. Administration of broad-spectrum or 'best-guess' intravenous antibiotics aid stabilisation of sepsis and the metabolic state prior to definitive treatment of foot sepsis by debridement or amputation will give the best result. Rarely, gas-forming organisms may be present; if gas gangrene is suspected, urgent surgery will be required after initial resuscitation.

## CASE SCENARIO 16.4

A 68-year-old, overweight woman was admitted in a coma. Her family provided a history of abdominal pain, anorexia and vomiting for 1 week against a background of 15 years of diabetes mellitus. In the early years, her diabetes was controlled by diet and oral hypoglycaemic agents; however, for the past 8 years, she had required subcutaneous insulin supplementation. She appeared to be dry and had a temperature of 38.3°C, a pulse of 130/min and systolic blood pressure of 80 mmHg. There was epigastric fullness and guarding and she had sighing respiration with a smell of acetone on her breath. A chest X-ray showed basal atelectasis. Blood results showed Hb 10.1 g/dl, WCC 19.5 x 10⁹/l, Na 152 mmol/l, K 6.7 mmol/l, HCO 15 mmol/l, Cl 100 mmol/l, Ur 22.5 mmol/l, Cr 85mmol/l, glucose 36 mmol/l. Her urine was strongly positive for ketones.

### WHAT IS THE MANAGEMENT OF THIS LADY?

Clearly, this is a complex clinical problem that cannot be managed in a general ward. However, again, the patient should be managed according to the CCrISP protocol with simultaneous immediate assessment and resuscitation. Although she probably has a surgical problem, she also has diabetic ketoacidosis (DKA) and this needs to be managed jointly with endocrinologists in an HDU or ICU, with continuous ECG monitoring and close biochemical monitoring of glucose (hourly) and potassium (3–4 hourly) levels (Tables 16.3 and 16.4).

## TABLE 16.4

### A POTASSIUM REPLACEMENT REGIMEN

In an unstable patient with varying insulin requirements, serum potassium levels should be monitored every 3–4 hours.

Replacement should be guided by the latest serum $K^+$ concentration
- if $K^+ > 5.0$ mmol/l, omit KCl due to the risk of cardiac arrhythmias
- if $K^+$ 3.5–5.0 mmol/l, add 20 mmol KCl to each litre of intravenous fluid
- if $K^+ < 3.5$ mmol/l, add 40 mmol KCl to each litre of intravenous fluid

DKA is uncontrolled hyperglycaemia with hyperketonaemia severe enough to cause metabolic acidosis. It is caused by severe insulin deficiency that stimulates lipolysis and a massive increase in ketogenesis. It is the hallmark of poorly treated type 1 diabetes but can occur in type 2 diabetes when patients are relatively insulin deficient and there is intercurrent illness stimulating counter regulatory hormone secretion (especially glucagon). It carries a mortality of 5–10% (50% in elderly patients with DKA precipitated by myocardial infarction or infection). Prompt diagnosis and management is essential to prevent death. As well as hyperglycaemia, hyperketonaemia occurs due to oxidation of free fatty acids (FFAs) in hepatocyte mitochondria (a process stimulated by glucagon and inhibited powerfully by insulin), yielding ATP and acetyl-CoA. The latter is converted to acetoacetate, which may be oxidised to 3-hydroxybutyrate or undergo condensation to produce acetone. Ketones are transported out of the liver and used as metabolic fuels by various tissues including the brain; they provide a few percent of the total energy needs after an overnight fast but this rises to one-third in prolonged fasting. When produced in excess, they accumulate rapidly as uptake mechanisms become saturated. The main consequences of raised circulating ketones are:
- acidosis, both extracellular and intracellular
- diuresis, as osmotically active ketones are filtered in the urine, exacerbating the osmotic diuresis caused by glycosuria, and resulting in polyuria, electrolyte losses, dehydration and hypovolaemia
- nausea – by direct stimulation of the chemoreceptor trigger zone in the medulla.

Simultaneous resuscitation and investigation includes a 12-lead ECG, bacteriological cultures of all appropriate fluids including blood and urine, cardiac enzyme determination and ABG analysis. Intravenous saline and insulin should begin immediately (Table 16.3). Urgent treatment with scrupulous clinical and biochemical monitoring is essential. Correction of hypovolaemia will often improve acidosis and hyperglycaemia. However, over energetic fluid and insulin replacement can predispose to cerebral oedema and increase mortality. CVP monitoring for the elderly and those at risk of heart failure is required. Monitoring for response is essential. 0.9% saline (with K when appropriate, see Table 16.4) is the fluid of choice. Dextrose 5% is substituted when plasma glucose has fallen to 10–14 mmol/l to prevent hypoglycaemia (insulin is still required to prevent ketogenesis and promote glucose utilisation in the tissues). Use of bicarbonate and hypotonic solutions is contentious; hypotonic solutions may exacerbate intracellular movement of water and could lead to cerebral oedema, while bicarbonate may improve extracellular acidosis; however, as membranes are not permeable to $HCO_3^-$ ions, the all important intracellular acidosis may not be improved. Indeed, $CO_2$ can enter the cells to combine with $H_2O$ to produce $H_2CO_3$ that can worsen intracellular acidosis with an adverse impact on outcome.

Hyperosmolar non-ketotic (HONK) state is distinguished from DKA by the absence of gross ketonaemia and metabolic acidosis. Hyperglycaemia may rise to higher levels but insulin levels are high enough to suppress ketogenesis. It is found in previously undiagnosed type 2 diabetes and may be precipitated by intercurrent illness, diabetogenic drugs (corticosteroids and thiazide diuretics) or fizzy glucose drinks. Complications include thrombotic events such as CVA, peripheral arterial occlusion, DVT and pulmonary embolism, due to increased blood viscosity. Mortality exceeds 30% because these patients are old and often have a serious precipitating illness. Lactic acidosis is generated rapidly during tissue anoxia (e.g. shock, cardiac failure or pneumonia) or when liver gluconeogenesis is impaired.

In diabetes mellitus, it is a rare, but fatal, complication of biguanides (phenformin, metformin), which act by inhibiting gluconeogenesis. It presents as coma with metabolic acidosis and a wide amino gap due to hyperlactataemia. Blood glucose levels are usually raised. Treatment is difficult: intravenous bicarbonate may aggravate intracellular acidosis; forced ventilation to blow off $CO_2$ may help; dialysis clears lactate and $H^+$ and will correct any sodium overload from bicarbonate infusion. Mortality is high (> 30%) because of co-existing organ failures.

# HYPOGLYCAEMIA

Hypoglycaemia is a dangerous side-effect of drugs that raise circulating insulin (i.e. insulin and sulphonylureas). It does not occur with dietary restriction, metformin or thiazolidinediones (e.g. roziglitazone). Common factors that predispose to hypoglycaemia are outlined in Table 16.5.

---

**TABLE 16.5**

COMMON FACTORS CONTRIBUTING TO HYPOGLYCAEMIA

**Accelerated insulin absorption**
- Exercise
- Hot environmental conditions

**Unfavourable factors relating to insulin administration**
- Too early
- Too much
- Inadequate food intake

**Alcohol consumption**
- Inhibits hepatic gluconeogenesis

**Impaired hypoglycaemic awareness**

**Diabetes control too 'tight'**

**Weight loss**

**Loss of counter-regulatory hormones**
- Addison's disease
- Hypothyroidism
- Hypopituitarism
- Blunted glucagon secretion (as in long-standing type 1 diabetes)
- Intestinal malabsorption
- Renal failure (impaired insulin clearance)

The events as blood glucose falls are listed in Table 16.6 but without early recognition can precipitate a coma. Hypoglycaemia should be recognised and treated immediately.

---

**PRACTICE POINT**

*Always remember to check the blood glucose with a BM stick in any patient with a reduced level of consciousness.*

---

**TABLE 16.6**

| CLINICAL EVENTS AS BLOOD GLUCOSE FALLS | |
| --- | --- |
| ~3.8 mmol/l | Adrenaline and glucagon secretion increases |
| ~3.0 mmol/l | Onset of hypoglycaemic symptoms (note, hypoglycaemic unawareness in some patients) |
| ~2.8 mmol/l | Neuroglycopenia and cognitive impairment |
| < 1.0 mmol/l | Coma |

## OBESITY

Excessive body weight is an increasing problem in people of all ages in the UK. The reference scale for obesity is the BMI, where the BMI is given by weight (in kg)/height (in m$^2$).

The normal range for BMI is 20–25 kg/m$^2$. Obesity is defined as a greater than 20% increase over the ideal body weight, which equates to a BMI over 30 kg/m$^2$.

Obesity increases the likelihood of associated medical disorders including ischaemic heart disease (especially central obesity), hypertension, oesophageal reflux, diabetes, obstructive sleep apnoea, osteoarthrosis, gallstones, varicose veins and haemorrhoids.

Reaching a diagnosis is often rendered more difficult. General anaesthesia and surgical procedures are more hazardous and postoperative complications, especially those relating to cardiopulmonary events, venous thrombo-embolism and the wound, are more frequent.

For elective surgery in non-life threatening conditions, pre-operative weight loss should be recommended. For all operations, a minimum of a blood glucose and ECG should be checked pre-operatively. Further investigations and pre-operative optimisation will depend on other patient and surgical factors. Proceeding to elective surgery requires a balance of risk versus benefit and may require careful discussion with the patient.

## ELDERLY

A social definition of elderly includes all those over 65 years of age and this group comprises about 1 in 4 patients admitted to surgical wards. Increasingly, patients over 80 years of age are being considered for major surgery and these patients provide a special challenge.

Two main reasons for increased risk with ageing are the frequent association of age and concurrent medical problems and decreasing functional reserve in many organ systems making the elderly less able to respond to the physiological consequences of operation. This is especially true for the respiratory system, cardiovascular system, kidneys, nervous system and drug handling. Again, careful assessment, optimisation and peri-operative care should reduce the surgical risk.

## RISK ASSESSMENT

Defining levels of risk to patients is important, both for enhancing the outcome of surgical intervention, and for managing the expectations of patients, their relatives and our colleagues. Verbal and written communication are vital to the management of expectation in these groups because there is a general perception that poor communication by surgeons may hide poor performance.

Assessment of clinical risk is a complex higher function to which all doctors aspire and which forms an integral part of training. Apart from direct clinical experience, how can we improve our risk assessment?

Evidence-based medicine provides different levels of confidence about the outcome of an intervention when examining published results. The most robust evidence comes from randomised controlled trials (RCTs) and meta-analyses of several RCTs on the same topic, while case-controlled series provide lower levels of evidence and case reports provide the lowest (but not always insignificant) form of evidence. These data often suffer from the constraints of carefully conducted trials but can be used in one's own practice to establish criteria for audit. Audit aims to improve the care of patients by establishing a standard, identification of areas for improvement and implementing that improvement, then evaluating the effects of implementation. Audit can also be national with contribution of data to national databases that are being established by the surgical specialty associations.

In the work place, mortality and morbidity conferences provide a forum in which factors that have contributed to adverse outcomes can be debated and strategies may be developed to improve unit outcomes. National surveys such as NCEPOD (National Confidential Enquiry into Patient Outcome and Death) allow panels of experts to analyse surgical deaths and make conclusions about their causes and recommendations for prevention. This can be around pre-operative preparation, the grade and seniority of staff involved and the resources available for treatment (*e.g.* NCEPOD theatres, ICU and HDU).

Measurement of risk aims to provide some objective evaluation of individual patient risk and can allow comparison of individual clinicians or units. This is fertile soil for research and a recent Medline search for surgical risk scoring revealed almost 1500 publications. Thus scoring systems have been developed in most subspecialties and for many individual conditions or procedures to try and produce a scale that will allow an accurate prediction of outcomes for each patient. Highly complex scoring systems may be unwieldy in the clinical situation and, when found to be valid in one unit or specialty, may require modification for successful adaptation to other specialties (*e.g.* the physiological and operative severity score for enumeration of mortality and morbidity, or POSSUM). Simple and more widely applicable scoring systems such as the ASA grading system is simple and in wide clinical use (Table 16.7). Most patients will be assigned an ASA grade (1–5) by the anaesthetist assessing the patient pre-operatively. Although simple and widely used, it is open to individual variation and even experienced anaesthetists may vary in their assessment of the same patient. This blunts its sensitivity and ability to discern actual risk for each patient.

**TABLE 16.7**

THE ASA SYSTEM FOR GRADING SURGICAL RISK

| Grade | Definition | Mortality (%) |
|---|---|---|
| I | Normal healthy individual | 0.05 |
| II | Mild systemic disease, does not limit activity | 0.4 |
| III | Severe systemic disease, limits activity but is not incapacitating | 4.5 |
| IV | Incapacitating systemic disease, constantly life-threatening | 25 |
| V | Moribund, not expected to survive 24 h with or without surgery | 50 |

Risk management is developing in healthcare and is borrowing ideas and techniques from the aviation industry that has practised risk avoidance with great success over many years. In addition to anticipating risk and the development of appropriate preventive strategies, a cultural change around the use of the information is required. Using adverse incident monitoring as an education tool, rather than one for apportioning blame, allows for learning appropriate lessons and putting strategies in place that minimise the likelihood of repeated failure. Also, aviation simulators that reproduce critical incidents allow important skills to be developed that can then be put into practice at appropriate moments when real lives are at stake. In surgery, this translates to the use of courses like CCrISP and skills laboratories in which clinical skills and techniques can be practised in the context of simulated patients and procedures in order that best practice can be learned and honed, for use in the clinical arena.

An international campaign to reduce harm in peri-operative care has led to initiatives such as 'Patient Safety First' within the NHS. This is based on an acknowledgement by healthcare workers that events that produce harm in patients are potentially avoidable. An example of one such initiative is that of reducing surgical site infections by establishing a target reduction and examining compliance with appropriate interventions to achieve it, including appropriate use of prophylactic antibiotics, maintaining normothermia, maintaining glycaemic control in diabetics and using recommended hair removal methods. In addition, to increase safety in the operating theatre, the use of the World Health Organization Surgical Safety Checklist is being piloted in hospitals. This is a 'time-out' before surgery (degree of urgency permitting); at the end of the procedure prior to transfer to the recovery area, the anaesthetist, surgeon, scrub nurse and other theatre staff discuss the patient preparation and any anticipated critical moments or potential complications and how these will be managed.

As champions for risk management, surgeons can demonstrate leadership in the care of patients that will improve the outcome of our treatment and operations.

## SUMMARY
- it is essential to recognise the factors that contribute to surgical risk
- ensure patients are as fit as possible prior to surgery
- be aware of co-morbidities to predict and prevent peri-operative problems
- manage diabetes carefully and precisely in the peri-operative period.

# INDEX